C Diff Colitis Demystified: Doctor's Secret Guide

Dr. Ankita Kashyap and Prof. Krishna N. Sharma

Published by Virtued Press, 2024.

C DIFF COLITIS DEMYSTIFIED: DOCTOR'S SECRET GUIDE

First edition. January 2, 2024.

Copyright © 2024 Dr. Ankita Kashyap and Prof. Krishna N. Sharma.

ISBN: 979-8224835683

Written by Dr. Ankita Kashyap and Prof. Krishna N. Sharma.

Table of Contents

DISCLAIMER

The information provided in this book is intended for general informational purposes only. The content is not meant to substitute professional medical advice, diagnosis, or treatment. Always consult with a qualified healthcare provider before making any changes to your management plan or healthcare regimen.

While every effort has been made to ensure the accuracy and completeness of the information presented, the author and publisher do not assume any responsibility for errors, omissions, or potential misinterpretations of the content. Individual responses to management strategies may vary, and what works for one person might not be suitable for another.

The book does not endorse any specific medical treatments, products, or services. Readers are encouraged to seek guidance from their healthcare providers to determine the most appropriate approaches for their unique medical conditions and needs.

Any external links or resources provided in the book are for convenience and informational purposes only. The author and publisher do not have control over the content or availability of these external sources and do not endorse or guarantee the accuracy of such information. Readers are advised to exercise caution and use their judgment when applying the information provided in this book to their own situations. The author and publisher disclaim any liability for any direct, indirect, consequential, or other damages arising from the use of this book and its content.

By reading and using this book, readers acknowledge and accept the limitations and inherent risks associated with implementing the strategies, recommendations, and information contained herein. It is always recommended to consult a qualified healthcare professional for personalized medical advice and care.

Introduction

The term "C. Diff. Colitis" whispers its presence in hospital quiet corners, worrisome conversations between loved ones, and the terrified thoughts of people who have been diagnosed. It frequently leaves a path of bewilderment and concern in its wake. What is this illness that causes havoc in people's lives and makes them anxious? The solutions aren't always clear-cut, but they're waiting for you to find them in these pages.

Imagine, if you will, a world in which the mysteries surrounding medical diseases are cleared up, the anxieties that come with receiving a diagnosis are allayed, and the path to recovery is made brighter by the glow of knowledge and comprehension. You are about to enter a universe where C. diff. colitis is debunked and you, the reader, are given authority.

Do you or a loved one suffer from C. diff. colitis? Are you an inquisitive person who is ready to analyse the complexities of this condition? Alternatively, you might be a guiding light for a friend or relative while they go through recovery. This book is your comfort, your guide, and your ally, no matter what position you play.

As we set out on this trip, we'll cut through the layers of medical jargon to uncover the essential information in language that speaks to compassion and clarity. The curtain of mystery is pulled back in this instance, revealing the facts concerning C. diff. colitis in a way that is both clear and understandable.

You could wonder, what is the essence of this condition? Now let's get to the core of the issue. The bacterium Clostridium difficile, also referred to as C. diff, can produce symptoms ranging from moderate diarrhoea to severe colitis, which is an inflammation of the colon. It's a strong foe that flourishes when our natural gut flora is upset, which frequently happens after taking antibiotics.

Now, let us pause for a while before we go any further into these waters. Inhale deeply. Experience the power of knowledge as it transforms the unfamiliar into the known. You will discover the definition of C. diff. colitis as well as its effects on the physical, mental, and spiritual aspects of life in each chapter.

"How can one navigate through the challenges of such an ailment?" may be on your mind. You may be sure that there are many options available to you that are designed to provide you with a biopsychosocial hug. In addition to emphasising the medical parts of treatment, this holistic approach also incorporates the psychological and social strands that are essential for a whole healing picture.

Think of the biological battlefield, where probiotics and drugs act as barriers against the toxins produced by C. diff. Imagine the mental health space, where mindfulness exercises and support groups help people feel better. Imagine the social realm, where lobbying and education create a resilient community.

This book's chapters are each a treasure mine of answers, a lighthouse pointing the way through the mist of doubt. You'll find the information you need to comprehend the function of antibiotics, identify the early warning symptoms of infection, and investigate the exciting possibilities of faecal microbiota transplantation.

However, what about the psychological impact and the strain on one's mental state? Do not be alarmed; we also handle this. You will learn how to take care of your mind and spirit in these pages, and how to find comfort even in the middle of the storm. There are tales of success and tenacity exchanged, all of which serve as evidence of the inner strength that everyone of us possesses.

As a patient, a friend, or a caregiver, what steps can you take to stop this difficult condition from developing or coming back? The decisions we make on a daily basis—from what we eat to how clean our hands are—hold the keys to the solutions, which are easier to find than you may imagine.

You will find medical experts' expertise, firsthand accounts from those who have been there, and helpful tips to strengthen your defences against C. difficile colitis in the upcoming chapters. We will examine the most recent findings, dispel popular misconceptions, and provide you a solid understanding that will act as both your shield and your sword in this conflict.

Remember this as we wrap up this introduction: knowledge is the light that chases away the darkness of uncertainty and fear. This book is more than just a collection of words; it is a source of hope, a companion on your path to wellness, and a guarantee that you are not alone.

Understanding C. Diff. Colitis

The Science Behind the Infection

The bacterium C. difficile, commonly referred to as C. diff., can produce symptoms ranging from diarrhoea to potentially fatal colon inflammation. Comprehending the intricacies of C. diff. colitis necessitates an understanding of its pathophysiology and microbiology. We will explore the complex mechanisms behind the onset and course of C. diff. colitis in this chapter, providing insight into the microbiological elements that contribute to its pathogenesis.

Understanding C. difficile's life cycle and habits is crucial to understanding the pathophysiology of C. diff. colitis. There are two different forms of this bacterium: spores and vegetative forms. The metabolically active condition known as the vegetative form allows the bacteria to proliferate and flourish inside the colon of the host. On the other hand, C. difficile may survive difficult environmental circumstances, such exposure to antibiotics or disinfectants, in its latent, robust spore form.

Spores of Candida difficile have the ability to colonise the colon and change into the vegetative form when they come into contact with a susceptible person. Toxins A and B, which the bacteria generates once it enters the vegetative state, are essential to the pathophysiology of C. diff. colitis. These toxins cause the intestinal epithelium of the host to malfunction normally, which results in inflammation and the telltale signs of an infection.

Changes to the gut microbiota are also part of the pathophysiology of C. diff. colitis. A diverse community of bacteria in the gut of healthy persons maintains a delicate balance. On the other hand, the natural gut microbiota is upset by antibiotic therapy, which fosters the growth of Clostridium difficile. As a result, C. difficile can become the dominant species in the gut and outcompete the native bacteria, worsening the infection.

Imagine that a patient is being treated for a respiratory infection with a course of broad-spectrum antibiotics. These medicines unintentionally upset the gut microbiota's delicate equilibrium, making the patient more vulnerable to C. difficile colonisation. The C. difficile spores germinate into the vegetative form and start generating toxins once they locate a suitable habitat in the stomach. As a result of this process, C. diff. colitis develops, which can cause severe diarrhoea, abdominal pain, and in extreme situations, pseudomembranous colitis.

Considering the viewpoints of the bacteria and the host is crucial for comprehending the pathophysiology and microbiology of C. diff. colitis. From the perspective of the bacterium, C. difficile's capacity to transition between spore and vegetative forms allows it to endure in the surroundings and settle in the host, guaranteeing its survival and spread. On the other hand, the host's vulnerability to contracting C. difficile infection is determined by a variety of circumstances, such as prior use of antibiotics, weakened immune system, and preexisting gastrointestinal disorders.

The incidence of C. diff. colitis has alarmingly increased in recent years, according to data from epidemiological research, placing a major strain on healthcare systems around the globe. Moreover, the genetic variety of C. difficile strains has been shown by genomic investigations, which have also illuminated the virulence determinants and antibiotic resistance profiles of these strains. These results highlight the complexity of C. diff. colitis and the difficulties in controlling and curing this infection.

Terms like "pseudomembranous colitis," "toxin-mediated inflammation," and "spore germination" may appear intimidating when discussing C. diff. colitis. To put these words simply, the production of inflammatory pseudomembranes in the colon—a defining feature of severe C. diff. colitis—is referred to as pseudomembranous colitis. The process by which C. difficile toxins cause an inflammatory response in the intestinal epithelium and contribute to the typical infection symptoms is known as "toxin-mediated inflammation." The process by which latent spores become active, metabolically functioning vegetative form of Candida difficile is known as spore germination.

In summary, the pathophysiology and microbiology of C. diff. colitis include intricate interactions between the host, the bacteria, and the microbiota in the gut. Deciphering the life cycle of C. difficile, the part toxins play in inflammation, and how antibiotic therapy affects the balance of gut microbiota are critical steps towards understanding the complexities of this infection. By thoroughly looking at these areas, we can learn more about the mechanisms of C. diff. colitis and develop better treatments, diagnostics, and preventative measures.

Diagnosis Procedures

This section aims to provide an overview of the medical methods and tests utilised in the diagnosis of C. diff. colitis. Through this exploration of the diagnostic procedure, readers will acquire a thorough comprehension of the actions required to detect and validate the existence of C. difficile in a patient, consequently enabling prompt and precise diagnosis and treatment.

Healthcare practitioners need access to some basic medical supplies and lab facilities in order to diagnose C. diff. colitis, including but not limited to:

1. relevant medical history of the patient, including symptoms related to the gastrointestinal tract and recent use of antibiotics.

2. Availability of a clinical laboratory with all the equipment required for the culture and analysis of stool samples.

3. Diagnostic instruments for identifying C. difficile toxins, such as enzyme immunoassays or polymerase chain reaction (PCR) testing.

4. To determine the severity of colitis, imaging tests such computed tomography (CT) scans or endoscopies could be required in specific circumstances.

A sequential strategy that includes laboratory tests, imaging examinations, and clinical evaluation is usually used to diagnose C. diff. colitis. First, a comprehensive evaluation of the patient's medical history and symptoms is conducted. Next, stool samples are collected and analysed to look for C. difficile toxins. It may be necessary to use other diagnostic techniques, such as PCR testing and imaging analyses, to determine the severity of colitis and confirm the existence of C. difficile.

Beginning with a thorough clinical examination of the patient, C. diff. colitis is diagnosed. Healthcare professionals obtain relevant data about the patient's past medical history, use of antibiotics recently, and symptoms related to the gastrointestinal tract. Particular focus is placed on signs of C. difficile infection, such as fever, stomach pain, and frequent diarrhoea. To further inform the diagnostic strategy, the existence of risk factors such immunosuppression, recent hospitalisation, or prior episodes of C. difficile infection is carefully evaluated.

Stool samples must be collected for laboratory investigation if a clinical assessment raises a suspicion of C. difficile infection. For the purpose of improving the sensitivity of diagnostic tests, multiple stool samples may be collected. To stop the deterioration of C. difficile spores or toxins, the specimens are gathered in sterile containers and sent right away to the lab.

A key factor in the diagnosis of C. diff. colitis is the laboratory. When stool samples are received, different diagnostic tests are used to find out if C. difficile toxins are present. The most widely used method for identifying toxins A and B generated by C. difficile is enzyme immunoassays (EIAs). These tests are reasonably priced and offer quick results. It is important to remember that false-negative results can happen and call for the use of other testing modalities for verification.

Molecular testing procedures, such polymerase chain reaction (PCR) assays, are used when traditional diagnostic tests produce equivocal results or when a high level of sensitivity and specificity is needed. PCR assays specifically target the genetic material of Clostridium difficile, making it possible to accurately identify the bacterium and its toxins in stool samples. When there is still a significant degree of clinical suspicion for C. difficile colitis despite negative EIA results, molecular testing is especially helpful in confirming the diagnosis.

Imaging investigations are not often necessary for the main diagnosis of C. diff. colitis, but they can be in some situations. Abdominal computed tomography (CT) scans can be used to determine the degree of colonic inflammation and rule out issues like toxic megacolon. Furthermore, in individuals with severe or complex colitis, endoscopic inspection of the colon, using techniques such as flexible sigmoidoscopy or colonoscopy, may be necessary to see the distinctive pseudomembranes and take biopsy samples for histological examination.

Share practical advice and cautionary suggestions.

- A high index of clinical suspicion is necessary for a prompt and correct diagnosis of C. diff. colitis, especially in individuals who have recently been exposed to antibiotics and exhibit gastrointestinal symptoms. It is imperative for healthcare providers to remain vigilant in detecting possible cases of C. difficile infection in order to swiftly undertake proper diagnostic treatments.

- Healthcare providers should consider the patient's clinical presentation and risk factors when interpreting diagnostic test results, as sensitivity and specificity might vary widely. If there is a strong clinical suspicion of C. diff. colitis, negative test findings shouldn't stop further investigation.

- To direct additional diagnostic and treatment approaches when preliminary diagnostic tests yield conflicting results or are inconsistent with the clinical picture, speaking with gastroenterologists or infectious disease specialists may be helpful.

Verification of the successful completion of the diagnostic process for C. diff. colitis is achieved by combining clinical, laboratory, and, if required, imaging results. When comparable clinical symptoms, positive C. difficile toxin laboratory results, and, if relevant, supportive imaging evidence align to indicate the presence of C. difficile infection and accompanying colitis, a definitive diagnosis is made.

Healthcare professionals should use caution when interpreting the results of first diagnostic tests that produce inconsistent or inconclusive results. They should also take into account the possibility that other testing modalities may be necessary to establish the diagnosis. Speaking with experts in infectious diseases or clinical microbiology can help in overcoming diagnostic obstacles and creating a diagnostic algorithm that is suitable for the specific clinical situation of each patient.

To sum up, the process of diagnosing C. diff. colitis involves a methodical approach that includes laboratory testing, clinical assessment, and sometimes imaging tests. A thorough comprehension of the sequential phases in the diagnosis of C. difficile infection is necessary to enable timely and accurate detection of this pathogen, which in turn allows for the timely implementation of targeted medication and infection control measures.

Risk Factors and Prevention

Risk Factors and Prevention of C. difficile Infection

A important infection linked to healthcare settings, C. difficile infection (CDI) is characterised by a range of clinical symptoms from asymptomatic colonisation to severe, life-threatening colitis. Reducing the prevalence of CDI and the morbidity and death that it causes requires an understanding of the risk factors that predispose people to the infection and the implementation of effective preventive strategies. The purpose of this part is to examine the preventive strategies that can lessen the spread and acquisition of C. difficile as well as to compare and contrast the risk factors for CDI.

This study aims to clarify the complex relationship between infection control practises, environmental factors, and individual susceptibility in order to provide insight into the intricate interplay between these variables. This analysis aims to give a thorough understanding of the drivers of CDI and the various approaches to its prevention by comparing and contrasting risk factors and prevention. This understanding will aid in the establishment of focused interventions and public health initiatives.

Risk Factors and Preventive Measures for CDI

The assessment of environmental variables, such as hospital facilities and community reservoirs, and the identification of individual-level risk factors, such as age, comorbidities, and antibiotic exposure, serve as benchmarks for comparison. The analysis will also take into account the effectiveness of vaccination, antimicrobial stewardship, and infection control procedures in halting the spread and acquisition of CDI.

Similarities in Risk Factors and Prevention of CDI

There are several parallels between the protective factors used to limit the spread of CDI and the risk factors for the disease. The importance of antibiotic exposure in the aetiology of CDI is highlighted by both of these factors. Moreover, the way that healthcare facilities contribute to the spread of CDI is also reflected in the preventive focus placed on infection control measures.

Nuances in Risk Factors and Prevention of CDI

Although the susceptibility to CDI is influenced by individual-level risk factors including advanced age and co-occurring illnesses, the preventive efforts go beyond individual interventions to include larger public health measures like immunisation campaigns and antibiotic stewardship programmes. Furthermore, the differences between CDI risk factors and prevention are rooted in the complexity of environmental reservoirs and the range of strategies needed to reduce transmission in healthcare and community environments.

Infographics and Epidemiological Maps

The reader's understanding of the intricate dynamics involved in CDI can be improved by making use of visual aids like infographics that show how risk factors and preventive measures interact, as well as epidemiological maps that show the geographic distribution of CDI incidence and the effects of preventive interventions.

Insights into CDI Risk Factors and Prevention

The examination of the risk variables associated with CDI offers significant understanding of the complex nature of susceptibility, emphasising the interaction of environmental reservoirs, microbial pathogenicity, and host factors. This knowledge emphasises the necessity of a thorough strategy for preventing CDI that takes into account public health initiatives, infection control procedures, antibiotic stewardship, and individual risk factors.

Contemporary Relevance of CDI Prevention

Effective preventive methods are still relevant in today's healthcare environment due to the rise in community-associated CDI and the introduction of hypervirulent strains of C. difficile. The development of vaccinations against C. difficile and the incorporation of novel therapies, such as faecal microbiota transplantation, highlight the dynamic character of CDI prevention and the continuous need for creative approaches.

The C. difficile infection, also known as CDI, is a complex infection linked to healthcare that presents a number of clinical problems to public health and healthcare systems. Mitigating the effects of CDI requires an understanding of the complex web of risk factors and the implementation of efficient preventive interventions. This section explores the intricate relationships between individual vulnerability, environmental factors, and infection control measures, providing insight into the complexity of CDI risk factors and prevention.

The pathophysiology and transmission of C. difficile are caused by a wide range of individual-level, microbial, and environmental variables that are included in the risk factors for CDI. At the individual level, the following stand out as major risk factors: a history of antibiotic exposure, comorbid diseases, and advanced age. Antimicrobial medication alters the gut microbiota, which increases the risk of infection by creating an ecological niche that is favourable to C. difficile colonisation and proliferation. Furthermore, worries about the seriousness and transmissibility of CDI have increased due to the appearance of hypervirulent strains like ribotype 027, which has increased the influence of microbial virulence on illness manifestation.

Apart from personal vulnerability, environmental reservoirs are essential for the spread of CDI. Due to the spores' longevity in the environment and the possibility of patient cross-contamination, healthcare settings—especially hospitals and long-term care facilities—act as hubs for the spread of C. difficile. In addition, the complexities of CDI epidemiology and the difficulties in stopping the dynamics of transmission are exacerbated by the community reservoirs of C. difficile, which include asymptomatic carriers and environmental pollution.

Effective CDI prevention strategies use a multimodal approach to addressing the complex network of risk factors and transmission channels. Antimicrobial stewardship initiatives, which maximise the prudent use of antibiotics, reduce needless exposure, and maintain the ecological balance of the gut microbiota, are essential to the mitigation of CDI. Using evidence-based infection control measures, such as hand washing, cleaning the environment, and taking contact precautions, is essential to stopping the nosocomial transmission of C. difficile and reducing outbreaks linked to healthcare.

Public health campaigns and community-based interventions, in addition to individual interventions and healthcare settings, are crucial in addressing the wider epidemiology of CDI. Immunocompromised patients and the elderly are examples of high-risk populations for vaccination techniques that show promise in lowering the incidence of CDI and averting serious illness consequences. In addition, the investigation of new treatments, including transplanting faccal microbiota, offers creative paths toward the restoration of gut microbial diversity and the prevention of recurrent CDI.

The dynamic nature of healthcare-associated infections and the constant challenges given by the evolution of C. difficile strains characterise the current landscape of CDI prevention. Strong preventative efforts are still relevant in the modern day due to the rise of hypervirulent strains, the influence of antibiotic resistance, and the rising prevalence of community-associated CDI. The introduction of new treatments, such as vaccines and monoclonal antibodies that target C. difficile toxins, highlights how CDI prevention is changing and how creative approaches are needed to defeat this dangerous infection.

In summary, the intricacy of C. difficile infection goes beyond its clinical presentation to include the complex network of risk factors that contribute to susceptibility and the variety of preventative actions that are crucial to reducing its spread. This research sheds light on how microbial, environmental, and individual-level factors are interrelated, which is helpful in understanding the complex nature of CDI and the range of strategies needed to lessen its effects.

The creation of focused therapies and public health campaigns intended at lessening the burden of this infection and enhancing patient outcomes are built upon the analysis of CDI risk factors and prevention. The C. difficile infection poses challenging problems that require continued study of creative preventative measures and integration of evidence-based interventions as the landscape of healthcare-associated infections continues to change.

The finished section offers a thorough examination of the risk factors for C. difficile infection and the precautions that are necessary to lessen its effects. The risk variables and prevention techniques that are compared and contrasted provide important insights into the complex nature of CDI and the range of strategies needed to tackle this tough infection. The formal language and intellectual tone preserve academic rigour and clarity, guaranteeing the section's appropriateness within the book.

Complications and Comorbidities

In order to fully address the impact of this formidable bacterium, it is imperative to explore potential consequences and associated health disorders as knowledge about C. difficile infection (CDI) and preventive strategies grows. In order to shed light on the complicated nature of the consequences that can result from a C. difficile infection and the connections with different health conditions, this section will explore the intricacies of CDI-related complications and comorbidities.

The main problem with CDI-related complications and comorbidities is the wide range of consequences that can result from an infection with C. difficile, from minor gastrointestinal problems to serious, life-threatening symptoms. The intricacy of CDI-related problems and their potential to worsen existing medical disorders are attributed to the interaction between C. difficile and its effects on the gut microbiota, host immune response, and systemic inflammation.

Untreated CDI-related sequelae and comorbidities have a variety of negative effects on public health, the economy, and therapeutic practise. These comprise the aggravation of pre-existing comorbidities, such as immunosuppression and inflammatory bowel disease, the chance of recurrent CDI, the possibility of chronic gastrointestinal dysfunction, and the financial strain on healthcare systems as a result of extended hospital stays and related expenses.

A holistic approach is necessary to address the complex problem of CDI-related complications and comorbidities. This approach should include the integration of preventive measures to reduce the impact of comorbid conditions on CDI outcomes, the optimization of supportive care for affected individuals, and the targeted management of CDI sequelae.

A multidisciplinary strategy comprising gastroenterologists, infectious disease experts, critical care physicians, and allied healthcare professionals is required to adopt strategies to manage CDI-related problems and comorbidities. The effective implementation of methods to reduce the consequences of C. difficile infection depends on the prompt detection of difficulties related to CDI, the proactive management of concomitant diseases, and the application of evidence-based interventions.

It is expected that the effective management of CDI-related complications and comorbidities will result in positive results, such as lower rates of recurrent CDI, better control over comorbid disorders, and the possibility of improved patient outcomes and quality of life. Additionally, it is anticipated that the incorporation of preventative interventions will help lower the morbidity and healthcare expenditures associated with CDI by lessening the influence of comorbid illnesses on CDI outcomes.

In order to mitigate the impact of CDI sequelae and their interactions with comorbid conditions, alternative approaches to address CDI-related complications and comorbidities may involve investigating novel therapeutic modalities, such as microbiota-targeted interventions and immunomodulatory therapies, to modulate the gut microbiota and immune response.

Beyond its clinical manifestations, C. difficile infection has many facets that cover a complex web of potential consequences and related health issues, emphasising the connection between CDI and different comorbidities. This section aims to give a thorough overview of the various ways needed to manage the impact of C. difficile infection on afflicted persons, as well as the sequelae that can result from the infection.

The range of complications associated with Clostridium difficile infection (C. difficile) includes a broad range of outcomes that may result from the interaction between C. difficile and the host, such as disruption of the gut microbiota, induction of inflammatory pathways, and the possibility of systemic symptoms. These complications range from mild gastrointestinal disturbances, such as diarrhea and abdominal discomfort, to severe, life-threatening manifestations, including toxic megacolon and sepsis. The impact of CDI sequelae on affected individuals underscores the need for targeted management and supportive care to mitigate their clinical impact.

The interconnectedness between CDI-related complications and various comorbid conditions further complicates the clinical landscape, amplifying the impact of C. difficile infection on affected individuals. Individuals with underlying inflammatory bowel disease, immunosuppression, or critical illness are particularly vulnerable to the exacerbation of their comorbid conditions by CDI sequelae, leading to prolonged hospitalizations, increased healthcare-associated costs, and the potential for long-term gastrointestinal dysfunction. The recognition of this interconnectedness underscores the imperative for a comprehensive approach to address both CDI-related complications and their interactions with comorbid conditions.

The targeted management of CDI-related complications and their interconnectedness with comorbid conditions necessitates a multidisciplinary approach involving gastroenterologists, infectious disease specialists, critical care physicians, and allied healthcare professionals. Timely recognition of CDI sequelae, proactive management of comorbid conditions, and the institution of evidence-based interventions are integral to mitigating the clinical impact and systemic consequences of C. difficile infection.

In addition to targeted management, the integration of preventive measures to mitigate the impact of comorbid conditions on CDI outcomes is imperative in reducing the burden of C. difficile infection and its associated sequelae. This encompasses the optimization of antimicrobial stewardship programs to minimize unnecessary exposure to antibiotics, the enhancement of infection control practices to curtail CDI transmission, and the exploration of novel therapeutic modalities, such as microbiota-targeted interventions and immunomodulatory therapies, to modulate the gut microbiota and immune response.

The anticipated outcomes of the comprehensive approach to address CDI-related complications and comorbidities encompass reduced rates of recurrent CDI, improved management of comorbid conditions, and the potential for enhanced patient outcomes and quality of life. The successful implementation of strategies to mitigate the sequelae of C. difficile infection is projected to contribute to the reduction of CDI-associated morbidity, healthcare costs, and the overall burden of this formidable pathogen.

In conclusion, the exploration of CDI-related complications and comorbidities illuminates the interconnectedness between C. difficile infection and various health conditions, emphasizing the need for a comprehensive approach to address the impact of CDI sequelae on affected individuals. By integrating targeted management, proactive recognition of comorbid conditions, and the implementation of preventive measures, this analysis seeks to mitigate the clinical impact and systemic consequences of C. difficile infection, thereby improving patient outcomes and reducing the burden on healthcare systems.

Case Studies: Real-Life Scenarios

The infectious disease unit of a busy metropolitan hospital was full of bustle as the staff got ready to handle a case of C. difficile colitis that had developed serious complications. For the previous two years, the patient, 68-year-old retired teacher Mrs. Thompson, had been suffering from recurring bouts of C. difficile infection. Her illness had steadily become worse despite numerous rounds of antibiotic therapy and supportive care, resulting in crippling gastrointestinal symptoms and a major deterioration in her general health.

The main character in this case study, Mrs. Thompson, had a complicated medical history that included a previous diagnosis of inflammatory bowel disease and immune system damage from long-term corticosteroid therapy. In order to handle the complex issues presented by Mrs. Thompson's C. difficile colitis, a multidisciplinary team comprising gastroenterologists, critical care physicians, and allied healthcare workers was gathered by lead infectious disease specialist Dr. Ankita Kashyap.

The main problem in this case study was Mrs. Thompson's persistent C. difficile infection, which was made worse by the serious effects of CDI-related comorbidities on her already-existing inflammatory bowel illness and weakened immune system. Mrs. Thompson's condition has worsened despite vigorous antibiotic therapy and supportive care, presenting a serious risk to her long-term health and well-being.

The multidisciplinary team developed a comprehensive approach to address the complex challenge posed by Mrs. Thompson's case. This approach included the targeted management of C. difficile colitis sequelae, proactive recognition of comorbid conditions, and the integration of preventive measures to mitigate the impact of complications related to CDI. In order to address the recurrent C. difficile infection, the treatment strategy comprised a variety of cutting-edge therapeutic approaches, such as immunomodulatory medications and microbiota-targeted interventions, which were designed to modify the gut microbiota and immune response.

After the all-encompassing treatment plan was put into action, Mrs. Thompson's clinical course showed a notable improvement. Her severe gastrointestinal issues eventually disappeared, and her general health and quality of life significantly improved. Moreover, the effective handling of her C. difficile colitis and its related issues resulted in a significant decrease in the frequency of recurrent CDI and a notable improvement in her overall prognosis.

The case study of Mrs. Thompson provides valuable insights into the crucial need of a multidisciplinary approach in addressing the complex issues associated with C. difficile colitis and its sequelae. The successful mitigation of the clinical impact and systemic consequences of C. difficile infection was largely attributed to the effective integration of targeted management, proactive recognition of comorbid conditions, and novel therapeutic modalities. These findings highlight the effectiveness of a comprehensive approach in managing complex medical scenarios.

In this instance, visual aids such as immunomodulatory drug regimens, longitudinal clinical data charts, and microbiota profiling would be very helpful in improving comprehension of the complex treatment strategy used in Mrs. Thompson's case and its eventual outcomes.

In addition to demonstrating the effectiveness of a comprehensive strategy, Mrs. Thompson's successful management of her C. difficile colitis highlights the larger storey of preventing recurrent CDI and its related consequences. The relationship between C. difficile infection and different comorbid conditions is clarified by connecting the details of this case study to broader themes of creative therapeutic modalities and multidisciplinary management. This opens the door to improved patient outcomes and less strain on healthcare systems.

Considering the complex issues surrounding C. difficile colitis and its aftereffects, it is important to ask how the knowledge gained from Mrs. Thompson's case might be applied to improve the treatment of recurrent CDI and its effects on patients with co-occurring disorders. This provocative question encourages more discussion and investigation of creative approaches to the complex problem of C. difficile infection and its clinical implications.

To sum up, the case study of Mrs. Thompson's struggle with recurrent C. difficile colitis is a powerful illustration of the ability of a holistic approach to effectively address the intricacies of problems connected to CDI and their interactions with coexisting illnesses. This analysis aims to shed light on the potential for improved patient outcomes and the reduction of the overall burden of C. difficile infection by exploring the nuances of her case and the creative therapeutic modalities used. This will pave the way for a more comprehensive and successful approach to managing this formidable pathogen.

The Biopsychosocial Model and C. Diff. Colitis

Biological Aspects of Treatment

The management of C. diff. colitis is a varied and intricate process that frequently combines pharmaceutical and physical therapies. Comprehending the biological components of various therapeutic approaches is crucial to appreciating their effectiveness and possible influence on patients' welfare. This chapter will examine the biological bases of different treatment modalities and how they relate to the management of C. diff. colitis.

The usefulness of antibiotic therapy in treating C. diff colitis is the main assertion that needs to be investigated. In particular, we will examine how antibiotics can treat Clostridium difficile infections and balance the microbiota in the gut.

The mainstay of C. difficile colitis treatment is antibiotics, which are designed to specifically target and eradicate the pathogenic C. difficile bacteria. Among the most often recommended antibiotics for this purpose are vancomycin and metronidazole. These antibiotics function by interfering with C. difficile's cellular functions, which finally causes the bacteria to die and be expelled from the digestive system.

By interfering with C. difficile's DNA synthesis, the nitroimidazole antibiotic metronidazole has bactericidal action against the bacterium. It is frequently recommended as the first line of treatment for milder cases of C. diff. colitis because of its effectiveness. On the other hand, because of its wider range of activity against gram-positive bacteria, including C. difficile, vancomycin, a glycopeptide antibiotic, is saved for more serious situations.

The severity of the illness, the existence of aggravating conditions, and the patient's medical history all influence the choice of antibiotic therapy. To reduce the chance of repeat infections and the emergence of antibiotic resistance, the length of antibiotic therapy also needs to be carefully evaluated.

Antibiotics have been shown to be effective in treating C. diff colitis, although there have been worries expressed about their propensity to alter the natural gut microbiota. The overuse of broad-spectrum antibiotics can cause dysbiosis, a disorder marked by an imbalance in the gut's microbial population that can put people at risk for recurring C. difficile infections and other gastrointestinal issues.

It is critical to address these worries by stressing the significance of using antibiotics sparingly and taking into account alternative therapeutic options, such as faecal microbiota transplantation (FMT). To counteract C. difficile overgrowth and restore the microbial balance, functional microbiota transfer (FMT) entails introducing healthy donor faecal microbiota into the recipient's gastrointestinal tract. In recurrent and resistant instances of C. diff. colitis, this strategy has demonstrated encouraging outcomes, underscoring the potential of microbiota-targeted treatments in the treatment of this illness.

Apart from FMT, the potential role of probiotics and prebiotics as biological treatments in preventing and treating C. diff colitis has been studied. The potential of probiotics—live bacteria that, when given in sufficient quantities, provide health benefits—to alter gut microbiota and strengthen host defences against C. difficile has been investigated. Prebiotics are indigestible food ingredients that encourage the establishment of good gut flora. They may also provide protection against infection and colonisation by C. difficile.

To sum up, the treatment of C. difficile colitis from a biological perspective involves a diverse range of therapies, including microbiota-targeted methods and antibiotic therapy. Antibiotics are still the mainstay of treatment, but in order to maximise patient outcomes, it is important to carefully examine alternative and complementary medications due to their possible impact on the gut microbiota. Healthcare professionals can work toward a holistic and individualised strategy to managing C. diff. colitis by including evidence-based biological therapies, which will ultimately improve patient well-being and lessen the burden of recurrent infections.

The Psychological Journey

The difficulties of having C. diff. colitis are multifaceted and frequently disregarded, and they go beyond the illness's outward signs. The psychological effects of managing a long-term gastrointestinal illness can have a substantial impact on a person's resilience, quality of life, and mental health. In order to provide patients with C. diff. colitis with complete care, it is imperative to comprehend and address these psychosocial components.

The main problem at hand is the severe psychological toll that people with C. diff. colitis endure. This load includes a broad range of psychological difficulties, such as sadness, anxiety, social isolation, and low self-esteem. An intense sense of helplessness and mental distress can result from the symptoms' unrelenting nature, the uncertainty around illness flare-ups, and the disruptions to everyday activities.

Ignoring the psychological effects of C. diff colitis can increase the overall burden of the disease and lead to a series of unfavourable consequences. A patient's mental health may deteriorate, which could hinder their ability to cope, lower their adherence to therapy, and affect how well they respond to therapeutic therapies. Moreover, the psychological distress may hinder patients' capacity to participate in social events, seek employment, and uphold significant connections, so jeopardising their general standard of living.

A comprehensive approach that incorporates psychological therapies alongside medical care is necessary to address the psychosocial problems associated with C. diff. colitis. Cognitive-behavioral therapy, mindfulness-based therapies, and psychosocial support are potential approaches to improve patients' psychological resilience and lessen the negative effects of the illness on their mental health.

In order to provide psychological support, mental health specialists like psychologists and psychiatrists must be included in the multidisciplinary care team for patients with C. diff. colitis. In order to maximise treatment programmes that take into account the psychological aspects of the condition, these specialists can interact with gastroenterologists, give individual or group therapy sessions, and provide customised psychological examinations.

Patients with C. diff. colitis can get cognitive-behavioral therapy (CBT) specifically geared to address their psychological needs. With the help of cognitive behavioural therapy (CBT), patients can better negotiate the psychological intricacies of their illness by recognising and altering maladaptive thought patterns, controlling anxiety-related symptoms, and developing coping mechanisms.

Mindfulness-based therapies, like as stress-reduction methods and mindfulness meditation, can provide patients with useful tools to help them cope with the emotional fluctuations that come with C. diff colitis. These therapies emphasise acceptance of challenging circumstances, present-moment mindfulness, and building inner resilience in the face of chronic illness.

Research has indicated that the inclusion of psychological interventions in the management of patients with gastrointestinal disorders that are chronic (such as IBS and IBD) might result in noticeable improvements in terms of psychological health, coping mechanisms, and overall quality of life. Similarly, it is expected that adding CBT, mindfulness-based therapies, and psychosocial support to the management of C. diff. colitis will have a favourable effect by enabling patients to better handle the psychological aspects of the illness and develop adaptive coping strategies.

Even if the suggested psychological interventions seem promising, it's important to recognise that complementary and alternative therapies may also be able to help people with C. diff. colitis maintain their psychological wellbeing. Additional possibilities for stress reduction and emotional control may be provided by relaxation techniques such as progressive muscle relaxation and guided visualisation. Additionally, combining expressive arts therapies—like music therapy and art therapy—can give patients a creative way to work with and express the emotional sensations they are having in relation to their illness.

In summary, treating the psychological aspects of having C. diff. colitis is an essential part of providing complete care for those who have this illness. Through acknowledging and addressing the psychological effects of the illness, medical professionals can enable patients to manage their condition with fortitude, vigour, and enhanced mental health. The holistic care of people with C. diff colitis can be optimised by including evidence-based psychosocial interventions and taking into account alternative supporting approaches, which will ultimately create increased patient empowerment and improved quality of life.

Social Support and Recovery

Living with C. diff. colitis is a complex and multidimensional experience that includes a deep psychological journey in addition to coping with the disease's physical symptoms. In this chapter, we explore the critical role that social support plays in the recuperation and overall health of people with C. diff. colitis. We will discuss the importance of having a strong support network, discuss how it may affect health outcomes, and offer doable tactics for maximising the benefits of social support for faster healing. In addition, we will discuss how social support treatments are put into practise and present previous or anticipated results to highlight how effective these strategies are at easing the psychological and physical symptoms of C. diff. colitis.

In the context of C. diff colitis, social support refers to the web of personal connections that include friends, family, medical professionals, and local resources. These relationships provide individuals navigating the intricacies of the illness with emotional support, practical help, and validation. The notion that managing a chronic illness requires a multimodal strategy that goes beyond medical therapies and includes the provision of psychological resources is the foundation for the provision of social support.

The main problem that emerges is the possibility that those suffering from C. diff. colitis may not receive enough or any social care at all. Lack of a strong support network can increase the psychological toll of the illness, which can result in more anxiety, less coping mechanisms, and a decreased ability to bounce back from a chronic illness. Furthermore, the absence of social support can lead to emotions of alienation, powerlessness, and isolation, which can make managing C. diff. colitis even more difficult.

In the context of C. diff colitis, the ramifications of insufficient social support are extensive and can have a significant influence on psychological health as well as disease management. People who lack a network of support may be more stressed, anxious, and depressed, which can make it difficult for them to manage their illness and take care of themselves. In addition, a lack of social support can cause a person to feel cut off from the outside world, which can lower their hope for recovery and degrade their quality of life.

In order to mitigate the lack of social support, a multimodal strategy involving the creation of networks of support, the development of interpersonal relationships, and the supply of community resources must be developed. Creating a supportive atmosphere that includes emotional validation, useful help, and compassionate understanding for people facing the challenges of C. diff. colitis is essential to maximising the impact of social support.

The execution of social support interventions necessitates a coordinated endeavour to mobilise diverse resources, such as healthcare establishments, patient support groups, and community organisations, in order to establish a favourable milieu for those impacted by C. diff. colitis. By incorporating the evaluation of social support into standard clinical care, healthcare providers contribute significantly to the creation of support networks by identifying patients who might benefit from focused interventions.

Social support is mostly reliant on the development of interpersonal relationships, thus people with C. diff colitis are advised to make the most of their current social networks, which include friends, family, and coworkers, in order to obtain both practical and emotional support. Additionally, patient support groups—both physical and virtual—provide a helpful forum for people to meet others going through comparable difficulties, exchange stories, and gain understanding of practical coping mechanisms.

Community resources that can help people with C. diff. colitis receive more social support include wellness programmes, peer mentorship programmes, and educational workshops. These materials provide those navigating the challenging landscape of chronic disease with a sense of empowerment, encouragement, and hope via the promotion of community and solidarity.

Empirical data has supported the effectiveness of social support therapies in improving the recovery and well-being of people with chronic illnesses, particularly gastrointestinal problems. Research has demonstrated the beneficial effects of social support on mental health, illness management, and quality of life, confirming its critical role in fostering adaptable coping mechanisms and resilience.

It is expected that the incorporation of social support therapies in the setting of C. diff colitis will result in observable advantages such as decreased psychological distress, more resources for coping, and better disease management. Through creating a supportive atmosphere that is marked by understanding empathy, helpful advice, and emotional affirmation, social support enables people to face the difficulties of C. diff colitis with more resiliency, optimism, and strength.

Although social support is a fundamental component of the all-encompassing care for patients with C. diff colitis, it is crucial to recognise the potential contribution of complementary techniques to enhancing the quality of social support. Relaxation methods, expressive arts therapy, and mind-body interventions are examples of complementary therapies that can be used as supplemental modalities to promote emotional resilience and well-being. These methods provide expressive ways for people to express their feelings, reduce stress, and develop inner resilience in the face of long-term sickness.

In summary, the provision of social support is a critical component of the comprehensive care that C. diff. colitis patients get. Through creating a supportive atmosphere that is marked by practical aid, sympathetic comprehension, and emotional affirmation, social support enables people to face the challenges of their illness with resiliency, bravery, and optimism. The holistic care of patients with C. diff colitis can be optimised by using evidence-based social support therapies and taking into account complementary techniques. This will ultimately promote increased patient empowerment and improved quality of life.

Integrating the Biopsychosocial Model

A complete framework that considers the interdependent effects of biological, psychological, and social elements on an individual's health and well-being is represented by the biopsychosocial model. The biopsychosocial model must be incorporated into the treatment strategy for C. diff colitis in order to address the complex and multidimensional nature of the illness. The objective of this chapter is to clarify the step-by-step process for incorporating the biopsychosocial model into the treatment of C. diff. colitis, assisting medical professionals and patients through each stage to attain the best possible results.

The main goal of incorporating the biopsychosocial model into the C. diff. colitis treatment plan is to promote a holistic approach that acknowledges the interaction of biological, psychological, and social factors in the development and treatment of the illness. By addressing the illness's psychological and social ramifications in addition to its physical symptoms, the aim is to enhance patient treatment and eventually promote overall wellbeing and better health outcomes.

Healthcare providers must have a thorough awareness of the biological foundations of C. difficile colitis, including its pathophysiology, clinical symptoms, and evidence-based medical therapies, in order to effectively incorporate the biopsychosocial model into the treatment strategy. To address the psychological components of the condition, competence in psychological assessment and therapeutic techniques is also essential. Furthermore, creating a supportive atmosphere for those suffering from C. diff. colitis depends on the availability of social support resources and community networks.

The biopsychosocial model is incorporated into the C. diff. colitis treatment plan through a thorough examination that covers the disease's biological, psychological, and social aspects. The basis for creating a customised treatment plan that attends to the various needs of people with C. diff. colitis is this assessment. For this reason, it is critical to apply evidence-based interventions across the biological, psychological, and social domains in order to achieve holistic care and encourage the best possible health results.

1. Biological Assessment and Intervention:

- Perform a comprehensive assessment of the biological variables influencing the development and presentation of C. diff. colitis, encompassing laboratory research, imaging analyses, and microbiological testing.

- Customize medical treatments, such as faecal microbiota transplantation and antibiotic therapy, to address the disease's biological symptoms and lessen the effect it has on the patient's health.

2. Psychological Assessment and Intervention:

- Use proven evaluation instruments to examine the psychological health of people with C. diff. colitis, including quality of life, anxiety, and depression assessments.

Use psychological therapies to improve coping mechanisms and treat the psychological impact of the illness, such as cognitive-behavioral therapy and mindfulness-based stress reduction.

3. Social Assessment and Intervention:

Evaluate the resources and social support systems accessible to people with C. diff. colitis, noting any weak points and any support gaps.

- Encourage participation in peer mentoring programmes, support groups, and community services to help people feel less alone and more socially engaged. This is especially important for those impacted by chronic disease.

- Tip:In order to provide a unified and integrated approach to patient treatment, encourage interdisciplinary collaboration among healthcare professionals, such as psychologists, social workers, and gastroenterologists.

- Tip:Stress the value of patient empowerment and education in assisting patients in navigating the complexity of C. diff. colitis and encouraging them to take an active role in their treatment and self-care regimens.

- Caution: Be mindful of the possible stigma and misunderstandings related to C. diff. colitis, as these may prevent people from getting the help they need and having honest conversations about their condition.

Comprehensive outcome measurements that cover the biological, psychological, and social domains can be used to validate the effective incorporation of the biopsychosocial model into the C. diff. colitis treatment plan. Assessments of illness remission, psychological health, social functioning, and quality of life are a few examples of these metrics, which offer a comprehensive analysis of the integrated approach's efficacy.

Healthcare professionals should be ready to address potential obstacles, such as resistance to interdisciplinary collaboration, limited access to psychological services, or insufficient social support resources, should difficulties arise during the integration of the biopsychosocial model into the treatment plan. Advocating for the inclusion of mental health services in the standard of care for C. diff colitis, developing partnerships with community organisations to expand social support initiatives, and raising awareness and de-stigmatizing the disease in healthcare settings and the general public are some strategies for overcoming these obstacles.

To sum up, the incorporation of the biopsychosocial model into the C. diff. colitis treatment regimen is a critical step in enhancing patient care and promoting overall wellness. Healthcare practitioners may provide comprehensive assistance to patients affected with C. diff. colitis by methodically addressing the biological, psychological, and social aspects of the disease. This approach eventually paves the path for improved health outcomes and enhanced quality of life.

Success Stories: Holistic Recovery

My approach to treating patients with C. diff colitis, as a physician and health and wellness coach, is based on a thorough biopsychosocial model that takes into account the interrelated effects of biological, psychological, and social aspects on an individual's health and well-being. I'm excited to offer success examples of patients who have healed by employing the biopsychosocial approach in this chapter, as this approach is intended to address the complex and multifaceted character of the disease. These narratives will offer an in-depth analysis of particular cases, highlighting obstacles, solutions, and outcomes in order to extract more general lessons and stimulate additional participation. The principal objective is to provide guidance and inspiration to those afflicted with C. diff. colitis as well as healthcare professionals, assisting them at every stage of the treatment process to ensure the best possible results.

Allow me to take you on a tour through the lives of those who have triumphantly overcome the difficulties posed by C. difficile colitis. These success stories demonstrate the effectiveness of the biopsychosocial approach in fostering comprehensive healing and changing people's lives. We can learn a great deal about the effectiveness of treating the disease's medical, psychological, and social aspects in order to accomplish complete healing by carefully examining the specifics of these situations.

Let us introduce you to Jane, a 42-year-old woman who has struggled for a number of years with the crippling consequences of C. diff. colitis. Her symptoms remained despite receiving a variety of medical treatments, including several courses of antibiotics, which had a detrimental effect on her quality of life. Moreover, the psychological impact of a long-term medical condition had resulted in emotions of loneliness and hopelessness. In addition to Jane, we will explore the experiences of Mark, a 55-year-old man who experienced comparable problems with C. diff. colitis and was able to restore his health and energy by using our holistic approach.

The main issue that both Jane and Mark had to deal with was the recurrent and chronic nature of C. diff colitis, which not only caused crippling physical symptoms but also had a negative impact on their mental health. Due to the limited effectiveness of standard medical therapies, a more thorough and integrative approach was required to address the intricate interplay of factors that contribute to the disease.

We used a customised treatment plan that included social, psychological, and biological interventions in our approach to treating Jane and Mark. In order to obtain insight into the underlying mechanisms causing the disease, we started by performing a thorough biological examination. This involved extensive microbiological testing, imaging scans, and laboratory investigations. These results led us to customise medical treatments, such as targeted antibiotic medication and individualised dietary changes, with the goal of reestablishing the gut microbiota's equilibrium.

At the same time, we acknowledged the significant psychological effects of long-term sickness on each of them. In order to address this, we evaluated their mental health using approved psychological evaluation instruments, identifying distressing regions and poor coping mechanisms. We then put psychological therapies into practise, such mindfulness-based stress reduction and cognitive-behavioral therapy, to provide them useful coping mechanisms and build their general resilience.

We also acknowledged the significance of social support in the healing process. Access to community services and support groups was made available to both Jane and Mark, which helped them feel less alone and more connected to others who are dealing with chronic illnesses. The goal of this multipronged strategy was to foster an environment that supported their general well-being.

Our comprehensive approach produced nothing less than extraordinary results. Jane, who had previously battled repeated bouts of C. diff. colitis, saw a notable improvement in her general quality of life in addition to a notable decrease in symptoms. She credited her recovery to the all-encompassing care she got, saying it made her feel more confident and in charge of her health. Mark also experienced a significant improvement in his quality of life, as evidenced by a reduction in both the frequency and intensity of his symptoms. The biopsychosocial approach's comprehensiveness had not only lessened the disease's physical burden but also given him the tools he needed to deal with the psychological and social difficulties that came with having C. diff. colitis.

The triumphs of Jane and Mark highlight how crucial the biopsychosocial paradigm is to fostering a comprehensive recovery from C. diff. colitis. Through coordinated approaches to the biological, psychological, and social elements of the condition, we were able to promote comprehensive healing that went beyond the conventional emphasis on symptom control. These examples demonstrate the transforming power of an integrated approach and provide insights into the intricate interactions between variables that affect health outcomes.

Figure 1 shows how Jane's and Mark's gut microbiota diversity changed after receiving individualised antimicrobial medication and making dietary changes. The correlation between the improvement in clinical symptoms and the enhanced microbial richness and variety after therapy underscores the relationship between biological interventions and overall health outcomes.

The success stories of Jane and Mark serve as an example of the larger storey of how a holistic and integrative approach can enable those impacted by chronic illness to regain their health and well-being. These cases highlight the importance of understanding how biological, psychological, and social elements interact to shape health outcomes and call for a move away from traditional medical intervention silos and toward comprehensive care.

As we rejoice in Jane and Mark's victories, we should also think about how the biopsychosocial approach can change the way that people with C. diff. colitis and many other chronic illnesses are treated. How might the power of integrative treatment be further harnessed to empower people on their path to recovery and to promote overall well-being?

In conclusion, Jane and Mark's success stories demonstrate the biopsychosocial approach's transforming power in fostering a comprehensive recovery from C. diff. colitis. Through analysing the subtleties of these situations, we have discovered the significant influence of addressing the disease's medical, psychological, and social aspects in a coordinated way, providing insights that go beyond conventional healthcare paradigms. These tales provide us rays of hope as we continue to negotiate the difficulties associated with long-term sickness, showing the way to full recovery and improved wellbeing.

Challenges in Holistic Treatment

As we continue to explore the intricacies of treating C. diff. colitis with a holistic approach, we come into a number of obstacles that may prevent the smooth execution of a treatment plan this extensive. This chapter will examine the challenges associated with combining social, psychological, and biological interventions and how these challenges may affect the holistic approach's overall efficacy. In addition, we will provide workable approaches and methods to overcome these obstacles, basing our suggestions on evidence-based analysis and anticipated results.

With a growing understanding of the interdependent effects of biological, psychological, and social factors on an individual's health and well-being, the healthcare landscape is changing. The incorporation of holistic techniques in the treatment of complex illnesses like C. diff. colitis has been made possible by this paradigm shift. But when we set out on this revolutionary path toward all-encompassing care, we encounter formidable challenges that need for thoughtful analysis and calculated manoeuvring.

The complex and diverse nature of C. diff colitis presents a number of obstacles to the implementation of an all-encompassing treatment approach. C. Dysbiosis of the gut microbiota is the hallmark of Diff. colitis, resulting in recurrent and incapacitating symptoms that damage the affected people's physical and mental health. Many obstacles may stand in the way of a coordinated and integrative approach that is necessary to address this intricate interaction of biological, psychological, and social elements.

Patients may suffer serious consequences if the difficulties in putting into practise a comprehensive treatment strategy for C. diff colitis are not addressed. In the absence of a thorough strategy that takes into account every aspect of the illness, people may endure protracted agony, reduced quality of life, and chronic symptoms.

Furthermore, the persistence of the dysbiotic state may be facilitated by ineffective holistic therapies, which could result in repeated infections and long-term health issues.

In order to overcome the challenges associated with executing a comprehensive treatment plan for C. diff. colitis, a multimodal approach that tackles every aspect of the illness in a coordinated fashion is essential. This entails combining social services, psychological support, and biological therapies to provide a thorough treatment plan that takes into consideration the many needs of those who are impacted. Moreover, the utilisation of predictive modelling and evidence-based procedures helps direct the creation of efficient solutions to surmount these obstacles.

A comprehensive biological assessment that includes imaging examinations, laboratory investigations, and microbiological testing to clarify the underlying causes of C. diff colitis is the first step towards implementing a comprehensive treatment plan. The results suggest that individualised dietary changes and targeted antibiotic therapy can be used to help the gut flora return to balance. The psychological effects of the illness can be addressed concurrently with psychological evaluations and treatments including mindfulness-based stress reduction and cognitive-behavioral therapy. Furthermore, helping people with C. diff. colitis get access to support networks and neighbourhood services can give them the social support they need.

There is evidence and expected results to support the suggested solutions to the problems associated with putting into practise a comprehensive treatment strategy for C. diff. colitis. Prior research has evinced the effectiveness of integrated biological, psychological, and social therapies in fostering all-encompassing recovery and enhancing general well-being among patients with persistent ailments. We expect a decrease in the frequency and intensity of symptoms, an improvement in the quality of life, and an increase in resilience in those who are impacted by the coordinated integration of these components.

Even though the suggested fixes are in line with the concepts of all-inclusive care, it's important to recognise that there may be other ways to deal with the problems that arise from holistic treatment. Assessing the practicability and effectiveness of innovative therapies, including biofeedback treatment, faecal microbiota transplantation, or community-based wellness initiatives, can provide more opportunities to improve the overall care of C. diff colitis. These alternate approaches need more research in order to increase the range of tactics that can be employed to support all-encompassing healing.

To effectively address the complex issues associated with implementing a comprehensive treatment plan for C. diff colitis, it is imperative to acknowledge the interdependent influences of biological, psychological, and social factors and develop strategies that systematically address these dimensions. Overcoming the challenges and utilising evidence-based understandings and anticipated results will enable us to cultivate a revolutionary strategy that encourages all-encompassing recovery and gives people the tools they need to go forward with their recovery.

The Role of Healthcare Teams

As we commence the revolutionary process of executing a comprehensive treatment plan for C. diff colitis, it is critical to acknowledge the critical significance that a variety of healthcare providers play in guaranteeing all-encompassing care. The cooperation of multiple healthcare teams is necessary to handle the complexities of this multifaceted illness, incorporate social, psychological, and biological interventions, and coordinate a coordinated strategy that puts the overall health of those impacted first.

a. Due to their proficiency in the diagnosis and treatment of gastrointestinal problems, gastroenterologists are essential to the therapy of C. difficile colitis. Their comprehensive comprehension of the disease's pathophysiology allows them to create customised treatment regimens that involve faecal microbiota transplantation, antibiotic therapy, and handling of consequences including toxic megacolon. In addition, gastroenterologists work in tandem with other medical specialists to track the effectiveness of treatment and manage recurring infections, all of which contribute to the overall care of patients.

b. Experts in infectious diseases offer a unique perspective to the treatment of infectious diseases, such as C. diff. colitis. Their knowledge of infection control and antimicrobial stewardship is crucial for directing the proper use of antibiotics, reducing the chance of recurring infections, and putting plans in place to stop the spread of C. diff in hospital environments. Infectious disease experts support the comprehensive approach by working with gastroenterologists and infection control teams to address the biological aspects of the illness and encourage antibiotic stewardship to maximise treatment results.

c. It is impossible to overstate the psychological toll that C. diff colitis has on its sufferers, and treating the psychological components of this complicated illness requires the collaboration of clinical psychologists and psychiatrists. In order to treat the emotional distress, anxiety, and depression that may accompany chronic illnesses, these mental health specialists provide psychological evaluations, psychotherapy, and psychiatric therapies. Clinical psychologists and psychiatrists help people battling C. diff. colitis feel better overall and be more resilient by incorporating psychological support into the comprehensive treatment strategy. d. Dietitians and nutritionists are essential to the comprehensive therapy of C. diff colitis because they offer individualised dietary advice that promotes gut health and general wellbeing. They help to optimise the nutritional status of affected persons and address the dietary triggers and considerations related with C. diff. colitis through their experience in nutritional assessment, specific dietary adjustments, and the management of malnutrition. Nutritionists and dietitians enhance the holistic approach by combining dietary therapies that assist the restoration of gut microbiota balance in conjunction with gastroenterologists and other healthcare specialists.

e. As essential parts of the healthcare team, nurses and nurse practitioners offer patients with C. diff. colitis thorough care, patient education, and advocacy. Their responsibilities include keeping an eye on symptoms, delivering medication, organising treatment regimens, and providing patients and their families with crucial support. A patient-centered and coordinated approach to care is ensured by nurse practitioners' conduct of evaluations, provision of continuity of care, and assistance in the implementation of treatment plans in conjunction with other healthcare professionals, all of which add to the holistic management.

f. C. diff. colitis has a complex effect that goes beyond its medical and psychological aspects. Social workers must be involved in order to address the social determinants of health as well with the day-to-day difficulties that afflicted individuals must overcome. Socioeconomic workers help people access community services, navigate healthcare systems, address social determinants of health, and give psychological support to individuals and families. Social workers address the social determinants of health and build resilience in those who are impacted by injustice by fighting for social justice and equity.

g. By addressing the functional and physical elements of the disease and how it affects everyday activities, physical and occupational therapists are vital to the holistic management of C. diff colitis. Their proficiency in mobility, functional independence, and rehabilitation allows them to design customised therapies that enhance physical health and maximise functional ability. Through the incorporation of physical and occupational therapy into the comprehensive treatment regimen, these practitioners help patients with C. diff. colitis recover and become better members of society.

Testimonies from those impacted by the disease and factual data support the roles that various healthcare teams play in the comprehensive management of complex disorders like C. diff colitis. The significance of healthcare teams in addressing the biological, psychological, and social aspects of the disease is highlighted by research studies, clinical outcomes, and firsthand stories. This ultimately improves the overall treatment and well-being of persons afflicted by the condition.

Healthcare teams work together to manage C. diff. colitis holistically, going beyond theoretical frameworks to practical applications that improve affected patients' real-world experiences. Gastroenterologists, infectious disease specialists, clinical psychologists, nutritionists, nurses, social workers, and therapists all seamlessly integrate their expertise to create coordinated care plans, individualised interventions, and all-encompassing support systems that cater to the various needs of people struggling with the complications of C. diff colitis.

Now that we have moved from explaining the critical roles played by healthcare teams to managing C. diff. colitis holistically, it is clear that the cooperative synergy of several healthcare providers is essential to coordinating a treatment plan. The convergence of viewpoints, the smooth integration of skills, and the coordinated efforts of healthcare teams open the door to a transformative approach that puts the complete healing and well-being of impacted individuals first.

To sum up, healthcare teams play a vital and diverse role in the comprehensive management of C. diff. colitis. This includes coordinating the integration of biological, psychological, and social interventions. The multidisciplinary teams of gastroenterologists, infectious disease specialists, clinical psychologists, nutritionists, nurses, social workers, and therapists work together to coordinate a coordinated strategy that tackles the intricacies of the illness, improves overall treatment, and builds patient resilience. The transforming potential of a holistic therapy approach that prioritises the holistic well-being and rehabilitation of persons struggling with C. diff. colitis is highlighted by the essential contributions of varied healthcare providers.

Preventative Measures and Lifestyle Changes

Dietary Adjustments for Prevention

Setting the process's objective is crucial as we set out to learn about the dietary changes required for the prevention of C. diff. colitis. The main goal is to alter the diet in a way that lowers the chance of getting C. diff. colitis and improves gastrointestinal health in general. People can establish an environment in their guts that reduces the growth of C. difficile bacteria and promotes a balanced population of gut flora by implementing particular dietary modifications.

Prior to initiating dietary modifications aimed at preventing C. diff. colitis, it is crucial to take into account the person's present health status, any prior medical issues, and any dietary restrictions or allergies. It is advisable to seek advice from a trained dietician or healthcare expert to make sure that any dietary modifications are in line with the person's general health and wellbeing. Implementing the suggested dietary modifications will also depend on having access to a range of whole foods, such as fruits, vegetables, whole grains, lean meats, and healthy fats.

Dietary modifications to prevent C. diff colitis are multifaceted and include both the addition of foods that support a healthy gut environment and the removal of those that are known to cause symptoms. The first step is to comprehend the fundamentals of a gut-friendly diet and then put these ideas into practise by taking doable actions to incorporate them into regular eating routines.

1. Understanding the Principles of a Gut-Friendly Diet:

Consuming high-fiber foods like fruits, vegetables, and whole grains is the cornerstone of a diet that is healthy to the digestive tract. These foods supply prebiotics, which support a healthy gut microbiota by acting as fuel for good gut bacteria.

- Including foods that have undergone fermentation, such kefir, yoghurt, sauerkraut, and kimchi, can help maintain a healthy balance of gut flora by introducing probiotic bacteria into the gut.

- Refined sweets and processed meals can upset the balance of gut flora and encourage the growth of pathogens, such as C. difficile, therefore it's important to limit your consumption of them.

2. Implementing Practical Changes in Eating Habits:

- Stomach pain brought on by abrupt dietary changes can be avoided by gradually increasing the intake of foods high in fibre and drinking enough water.

- Meal planning that incorporates a range of vibrant fruits and vegetables guarantees a varied consumption of vital nutrients and antioxidants that promote gut health.

- Eating meals that include lean proteins and healthy fats along with whole grains instead of refined grains increases satiety and supports digestive wellness in general.

- Dietary adjustments should be made gradually since abrupt changes in the amount of dietary fibre consumed might cause bloating and other gastrointestinal distress. Over a few weeks, gradually increasing the amount of fibre you eat will allow your stomach to adjust.

- It's important to watch portion sizes and refrain from overindulging because consuming too much food might irritate the digestive tract and cause disruptions in gut function.

- In order to promote healthy digestion and avoid constipation, it is necessary to boost water consumption in addition to fibre intake.

People can track their general health and digestive health to confirm that dietary changes for the prevention of C. diff. colitis have been successfully implemented. Reduced bloating, more regular bowel movements, and more energy are examples of symptoms that may point to beneficial improvements in gut health. Furthermore, periodic evaluations and feedback from a healthcare professional can validate the effectiveness of the dietary modifications.

To sum up, the process of modifying diet to prevent C. diff. colitis entails a thorough comprehension of gut-friendly concepts, realistic application of dietary modifications, and continuous assessment of digestive health. People can take proactive actions to build an internal environment that supports gut health and lowers the risk of C. diff. colitis by adhering to the suggested dietary alterations and following the stated instructions.

Importance of Hygiene and Sanitation

Sanitation and hygiene are essential for stopping the spread of Clostridium difficile (C. diff) infections, especially in hospitals and public areas. Controlling the spread of this bacterium requires knowledge of and adherence to strict hygiene protocols. We will examine the ideas, methods, and evidence-based tactics that support successful infection prevention in this chapter as we examine the vital role that hygiene and sanitation play in the fight against C. diff infections.

The foundation of infection control and prevention is sanitation, which is described as the supply of clean circumstances to avoid disease, and hygiene, which is the practise of maintaining cleanliness to retain health. These concepts are especially important in the case of C. diff since the bacteria is spore-forming, which allows it to survive on a variety of surfaces and withstand common disinfection techniques. Comprehending the pathways of dissemination, such as coming into contact with polluted surfaces or the hands of healthcare personnel, emphasises how important it is to implement strict hygiene and sanitation protocols to stop the spread of C. diff.

Strict attention to hand hygiene guidelines is essential in healthcare institutions to lower the risk of C. diff transmission. Healthcare personnel are required to strictly adhere to handwashing protocols, using alcohol-based hand sanitizers or soap and water, especially before and after patient contact. Furthermore, to minimise the persistence of C. diff spores and avoid cross-contamination, surfaces, equipment, and patient care locations must be thoroughly cleaned and disinfected.

Promoting proper hygiene in communal settings is essential to stopping the spread of C. diff. This includes frequent hand washing with soap and water, especially after using the restroom and before handling food. Adequate disposal of faeces and contaminated materials, along with other proper sanitation practises, help to lessen environmental contamination and the risk of transmission.

Imagine that a patient with a C. diff infection is admitted to a medical facility. Healthcare personnel can successfully stop the bacteria from spreading by strictly adhering to hand hygiene protocols, maintaining a clean work environment, and wearing personal protective equipment as needed. Comparably, in a community context, teaching people about the significance of cleanliness and hygiene in averting gastrointestinal infections, such as C. diff, can result in better public health outcomes and a decrease in the burden of disease.

From the standpoint of public health, the application of sanitation and hygiene interventions goes beyond specific behaviours and includes more comprehensive tactics meant to lessen the spread of C. diff in many contexts. This include the use of evidence-based guidelines for environmental cleaning and disinfection, targeted education and training for healthcare workers and the public, and surveillance programmes to track infection rates.

The impact of sanitation and hygiene on the spread of C. diff is demonstrated by empirical studies. Improved hand hygiene compliance and environmental cleaning techniques have been linked to lower rates of C. diff infections related to healthcare, according to studies. Additionally, epidemiological statistics emphasise the need for comprehensive public health interventions to address environmental pollution and highlight the role that inadequate sanitation plays in contributing to community outbreaks of C. diff.

Terms like "fomite contamination," "contact transmission," and "sporicidal disinfection" are commonly used in the context of infection prevention. The term "contact transmission" describes the spread of infectious pathogens by direct or indirect touch between individuals. The term "fomite contamination" refers to the presence of infectious agents on surfaces or objects that could act as conduits for transmission. In order to stop the transmission of bacterial spores, such as those caused by C. diff, sporicidal disinfection is the use of chemicals that may kill spores.

In summary, the careful application of sanitation and hygiene measures is essential to stopping the spread of C. diff. The diligent implementation of these guidelines lowers the incidence of C. diff infections in both the community and clinical settings. Effective hygiene and sanitation practises can help mitigate the effects of C. diff. Together, we can promote education and awareness, integrate evidence-based strategies, and cultivate a culture of infection prevention.

In the context of preventing C. diff infections, the significance of cleanliness and hygiene cannot be emphasised, as this chapter has shown. In the future, stopping the spread of this hardy bacteria will still require incorporating these ideas into routine procedures and public health campaigns.

Exercise and Physical Health

Exercise and physical activity are essential for preserving general health and wellbeing. Regular physical activity has benefits for C. diff colitis that go beyond overall fitness and may have an impact on controlling and avoiding the condition. In the context of C. diff colitis, this chapter will examine the connection between physical health and exercise, reviewing the research and possible effects of exercise on the management and prevention of this difficult illness.

By enhancing gut health, lowering the risk of infection and recurrence, and strengthening the immune system, regular physical activity can help prevent and manage C. diff colitis.

Numerous health advantages of physical activity have been linked, one of which is improved immunological function. Exercise on a regular basis has been demonstrated to increase the production of T-cells and natural killer cells, two types of immune cells that are essential for protecting the body from infections. This immune-stimulating impact might be especially pertinent in the setting of C. diff colitis, since fighting the bacteria requires a strong immunological response.

Exercise has also been connected to changes in the gut microbiota, which is the varied community of bacteria that live in the gastrointestinal system. Regular exercise has been linked to a more healthy and diversified gut microbiome, which is linked to better gut health and a lower risk of gastrointestinal illnesses, according to studies. Given that C. diff disrupts the gut microbiota to cause colitis, exercise's ability to positively affect the makeup of gut microbes may be helpful in both managing and preventing the illness.

Exercise is clearly beneficial for immune system function and gut health, but it's crucial to recognise that too much or too strenuous exercise may have the opposite impact. Excessive exercise and overtraining can weaken the immune system and cause gastrointestinal issues, which can make a person more prone to infections and compromise gut health.

However, the overall advantages of regular, moderate physical activity should not be overshadowed by the possible drawbacks of overindulging in exercise. Exercise has been repeatedly linked to favourable health effects, such as enhanced immune function and gut microbial diversity, when done at the right intensity and duration. Consequently, taking part in physical activity responsibly is essential to realising its potential advantages in controlling and preventing C. diff colitis.

Additional evidence for the beneficial effects of exercise in both preventing and treating C. diff colitis comes from studies showing these effects can be achieved through strengthening the intestinal barrier, lowering inflammation, and improving overall metabolic health. Given that gut integrity impairment and inflammation are two of the main characteristics of colitis, these effects are pertinent in this context.

In summary, there is strong evidence to support the advantages of exercise in controlling and avoiding C. diff colitis. Frequent exercise can improve gut microbiota health, strengthen the immune system, and reduce inflammatory processes—all of which are important for both avoiding and treating the illness. But given that too much physical activity can have negative effects, it is imperative to stress the need of balanced, moderate exercise. Regular physical activity can potentially lower an individual's risk of C. diff colitis and improve their capacity to effectively manage the condition when incorporated within a holistic approach to health and fitness.

Stress Management Techniques

When it comes to C. diff colitis, stress management strategies are essential to the general health of those who are diagnosed with this difficult disease. Stress affects the immune system, intestinal health, and general quality of life in addition to making C. diff colitis symptoms worse. In order to help with the prevention and treatment of C. diff colitis, this chapter will explain a number of stress management strategies that can be useful in reducing the negative effects of stress on the illness.

Originating in traditional contemplative practises, mindfulness meditation has become well-known in contemporary medicine for its ability to effectively reduce stress. Developing present-moment awareness and accepting oneself without passing judgement on one's ideas and feelings are key components of this practise. The advantages of mindfulness meditation in lowering stress levels, promoting overall psychological well-being, and improving emotional control have been repeatedly shown by research. Mindfulness meditation can be especially helpful when it comes to C. diff colitis because it gives patients the tools they need to deal with the psychological and emotional difficulties that come with the illness. Stress has a negative impact on immune system and gastrointestinal health. Mindfulness meditation can mitigate this impact by promoting a state of peace and tranquilly.

Several scientific research have demonstrated the therapeutic benefits of mindfulness meditation for the reduction of stress. For instance, a meta-analysis found that mindfulness meditation therapies were linked to significant improvements in anxiety, depression, and general well-being. The meta-analysis was published in the Journal of the American Medical Association (JAMA) Internal Medicine. Moreover, testimonies from people dealing with long-term medical conditions—such as colitis—have demonstrated the revolutionary power of mindfulness meditation in reducing symptoms associated with stress and boosting resilience in the face of health obstacles.

Including mindfulness meditation in regular routines can be a very effective way for people who are struggling with the stress of Crohn's disease. A organised meditation programme might include easy techniques like body scans and mindful breathing exercises. Furthermore, programmes offering mindfulness-based stress reduction (MBSR), which integrate mindfulness meditation with cognitive methods, provide thorough frameworks for anyone who want to adopt this stress-reduction approach. People who regularly practise mindfulness meditation can build robust thought patterns and flexible coping strategies to deal with the challenges of having C. diff colitis.

Now that we have looked at the many advantages of mindfulness meditation for stress reduction, we will look at cognitive-behavioral therapy as the next stress-reduction strategy (CBT).

The goal-oriented, structured therapeutic technique known as cognitive-behavioral therapy (CBT) focuses on unhelpful thought and behaviour patterns that lead to stress and emotional suffering. The fundamental ideas of cognitive behavioural therapy (CBT) are around recognising and rephrasing harmful thought patterns, creating useful coping mechanisms, and encouraging behavioural changes that lead to enhanced mental health. When it comes to C. diff colitis, cognitive behavioural therapy (CBT) can be a useful technique for managing the psychological effects of the illness, including sadness, anxiety, and the emotional burden of a chronic illness. CBT shows promise in reducing the negative effects of stress on the development and treatment of C. diff colitis by providing people with the cognitive and behavioural tools they need to manage stress.

Research supports CBT's effectiveness in stress reduction for a variety of demographics. Research has indicated that Cognitive Behavioral Therapy (CBT) therapies result in noteworthy decreases in stress, anxiety, and depressive symptoms, along with long-lasting impacts on psychological resilience. Testimonials from patients receiving CBT for long-term medical illnesses further highlight how transformative this therapeutic approach is in improving coping mechanisms, regaining control, and reducing the psychological toll that comes with being sick.

Cognitive restructuring, behavioural activation, and relaxation training are examples of CBT strategies that can be customised to meet the unique pressures and emotional difficulties that people with C. diff colitis face. Practical uses of CBT that can help people manage the psychological effects of the disease include progressive exposure to stressors, confronting cognitive distortions, and self-monitoring of thoughts and emotions. Furthermore, incorporating cognitive behavioural therapy (CBT) into all-encompassing treatment regimens for C. diff colitis might increase the patient's ability to regulate stress, which will ultimately lead to better health and better disease control.

After discussing the therapeutic potential of cognitive behavioural therapy (CBT) for stress management, we will now examine exercise and physical activity as a stress management strategy.

Probiotics and Gut Health

The medical community is very interested in and conducting research on the function of probiotics in preserving gut health and avoiding colitis caused by C. diff. Probiotics are live bacteria that, when taken in sufficient quantities, offer health advantages. They have gained popularity due to their ability to alter the gut microbiota, support the immune system, and reduce the risk of C. diff colitis. This chapter aims to clarify the ways in which probiotics safeguard gut health, investigate the data pertaining to their application in the setting of C. diff colitis, and respond to any relevant drawbacks or objections.

The assertion that probiotic use is essential for preserving gut health and guards against C. diff colitis will be investigated.

Probiotics, which include a wide variety of bacterial strains like Lactobacillus, Bifidobacterium, and Saccharomyces, have been the subject of much research due to their potential to alter the gut microbiota's composition and function. Probiotics and the indigenous gut bacteria, referred to as the microbiome, have complex interactions that affect immune control, nutrition metabolism, and the preservation of the gut barrier. Probiotics, it should be noted, have been demonstrated to compete with pathogenic bacteria, such as C. difficile, for colonisation sites in the gut, preventing both their growth and harmful activity.

Probiotics are effective in preventing C. diff colitis, as evidenced by a number of studies that explain how they work. According to studies, some probiotic strains contain organic acids and antibacterial substances that make it difficult for C. difficile to colonise and produce toxins. Additionally, probiotics have been shown to improve the function of the gut barrier, strengthen mucosal immunity, and regulate inflammatory responses—all of which help to lessen the risk of developing C. diff colitis and other gastrointestinal diseases.

Probiotics have a lot of data supporting them, although different research have found different levels of probiotic therapies' efficacy in preventing C. diff colitis. Inconsistent results among clinical trials may be caused by variables like the particular probiotic strains utilised, their dosage, and the variety of patient populations. Personalized approaches to probiotic therapy are necessary because individual differences in the composition of their gut microbiota and host immunological responses may affect how well they respond to probiotic administration.

Owing to the fluctuations in probiotic effectiveness, current research efforts are concentrated on clarifying the elements that impact the effectiveness of probiotic treatments. The best probiotic formulations for reducing the risk of C. diff colitis are being researched based on strain-specific traits like immunomodulatory effects, metabolic activity, and adhesion properties. Probiotic regimens can be customised to each person's unique microbiota composition, enhancing their therapeutic potential, thanks to developments in personalised medicine and microbiome analysis.

Meta-analyses that compile the results of several clinical trials and preclinical research can provide more evidence for the benefit of probiotics in preserving gut health and reducing C. diff colitis. These sources offer thorough insights into the various mechanisms—such as the modification of host-microbiota interactions, the augmentation of barrier function, and the suppression of inflammatory cascades—through which probiotics maintain gut health.

To sum up, the data demonstrating the function of probiotics in preserving intestinal integrity and averting C. diff colitis highlights their potential as an important supplement to traditional treatment modalities. Although there are many complex factors that affect the effectiveness of probiotics, more investigation and tailored strategies may be able to improve probiotic usage in the setting of C. diff colitis. Adopting probiotics as the cornerstone of managing gut health indicates a proactive approach to strengthening the gut ecology and preventing the development and recurrence of C. diff colitis.

Travel Precautions

People who travel for work or pleasure are subjected to different food restrictions, changed circadian rhythms, and different environmental conditions. These variables may have a major effect on the delicate balance of the gut microbiota and may make people more susceptible to developing C. difficile (C. diff) colitis. Consequently, it becomes essential to provide travel advice in order to reduce the risk of C. diff colitis and to support gut health in general.

The main problem here is the increased vulnerability to C. diff colitis resulting from immune system and gut microbiota change during travel. Dietary modifications, exposure to foreign pathogens, and sleep disorders can weaken the gut's defences, which makes it easier for C. difficile to colonise and engage in pathogenic activity.

An increased incidence of C. diff colitis among travellers may result from a failure to address the difficulties provided by disturbances to gut health caused by travel. The ramifications could impair the general health and travel experience of those who are impacted, such as gastrointestinal distress, extended recuperation times, and the possibility of recurring infections.

It is advised to take a multimodal approach that includes dietary changes, good cleanliness, and the prudent use of probiotics as preventive measures to reduce the risk of C. diff colitis while travelling. In order to prevent the start of C. diff colitis while travelling, it can be prudent to prioritise the preservation of gut health through focused therapies.

A thorough travel health plan should include probiotic supplements to support gut resilience, dietary modifications to maintain gut microbial diversity, and strict attention to hygiene precautions to reduce pathogen exposure. Furthermore, the implementation of preventative measures, such as refraining from the needless use of antibiotics, and responsible antimicrobial stewardship play a critical role in preserving gut health when travelling.

Studies in the past have shown that those who take precautions when travelling have lower rates of gastrointestinal infections, such as C. diff colitis. By implementing focused measures to preserve gut health, the risk of acquiring C. difficile can be reduced by reducing the impact of travel-related disturbances on the immune system and gut microbiota.

Alternative strategies, such as the use of prebiotics, which act as substrates for beneficial gut bacteria, and the incorporation of particular dietary components with antimicrobial properties, may offer complementary avenues to fortify gut health during travel, even though the proposed approach prioritises dietary modifications, hygiene practises, and probiotic supplementation.

When tourists set out on adventures that cover a wide range of geographical locations, gastronomic delights, and differing levels of hygiene, the health of their digestive tracts becomes critical. Because travel-related disruptions can take many forms, protecting gut health and reducing the risk of C. diff colitis require a sophisticated strategy. Through the integration of proactive interventions and evidence-based tactics, people can effectively manage the difficulties associated with travel while maintaining the resilience of their gut environment. As such, the adoption of customised travel measures becomes an essential undertaking for the overall maintenance of intestinal health and the avoidance of C. diff colitis.

Personal Stories: Lifestyle Overhaul

I was standing outside Mrs. Evelyn Thompson's charming cottage as the sun was rising over the peaceful countryside, illuminating the wide swath of greenery with a warm glow. Her abode was peaceful and seemed to exist outside of time, even though it was surrounded by beautiful scenery. This was the tale of Mrs. Thompson, a woman who had a remarkable metamorphosis and managed to escape the grip of C. difficile (C. diff) colitis by adopting a more holistic way of living.

Freshly opened flowers mixed with the earthy perfume of the nearby woods floated through the air. The peaceful surroundings belied the turbulent journey Mrs. Thompson had made—a journey that would soon come to an end in front of my eyes.

Mrs. Thompson had a calm tenacity about her, resilience formed by unflinching determination seen in her eyes. Her voyage served as evidence of the unbreakable spirit she possessed, a spirit that had enabled her to overcome all the obstacles in her path.

Once I was comfortably seated in her living room, Mrs. Thompson started to narrate the incidents that had caused her life to fall apart. Her detailed account of her experiences with C. diff colitis, a malady that had threatened to destroy the fundamental fabric of her existence and cast a cloud over her well-being, was moving.

Mrs. Thompson's speech struck a profound chord with me because of how openly she described the anguish and hopelessness that had consumed her in the final stages of her sickness. I felt intense pity for her because I could see the toll it had taken on her mental and physical health.

When all hope appeared to be lost, Mrs. Thompson set out on a quest that would challenge accepted medical wisdom. She turned to holistic health care and wellness, which was a less-traveled route with the potential for healing and rejuvenation.

Mrs. Thompson's storey went beyond her own hardship and provided a deep understanding of the global fight against C. diff colitis. Her experiences demonstrated the human spirit's tenacity and the transformational potential of adopting a holistic perspective on health and wellbeing.

As the storey of Mrs. Thompson came to light, it was clear that there was a wealth of knowledge and understanding included in the account. Her experience provided evidence of the significant effects of dietary planning, holistic wellness, and lifestyle adjustments in overcoming the sneaky grasp of C. diff colitis.

Mrs. Thompson's journey began when the entangling tendrils of C. diff colitis had snagged her into an unending cycle of crippling symptoms and repeated infections. Although traditional medical treatments had provided a brief period of relief, the threat of recurrence remained large, putting doubt on her prospects. In search of a long-term fix, she navigated the unexplored territory of holistic treatment against this backdrop of hardship.

It was nothing short of amazing how things changed. Motivated by a solitary goal to restore her health, Mrs. Thompson adopted a multimodal strategy with the support of a committed group of health and wellness specialists, led by me, Dr. Ankita Kashyap. Together, we mapped out a course of action that included customised dietary adjustments, alternative and complementary therapies, and lifestyle modifications based on her particular requirements.

The foundation of Mrs. Thompson's journey was the painstaking formulation of a customised meal plan, which was carefully designed to support her body's natural defences and foster the diversity of her gut bacteria. She adopted a diet of complete, nutrient-dense foods and set out on a culinary journey to maximise the natural healing power of the abundant produce of nature. Every meal evolved into a harmonious blend of tastes and nutrients, with every component serving as evidence of the life-changing potential of mindful eating.

In addition, Mrs. Thompson engaged herself in a fabric of lifestyle adjustments that went beyond traditional medical paradigms. She created a haven of wellbeing that nourished her body, mind, and soul, from the warm embrace of holistic therapies to the restorative disciplines of mindfulness and self-care. This entire tapestry gave her a strong sense of empowerment and vigour, acting as a furnace for her perseverance.

Alongside these changes to her way of life, Mrs. Thompson started a voyage of self-discovery that allowed her to find her mind and spirit's untapped potential. She was able to unwind the knots of stress and anxiety that had tied her to the depths of disease by navigating the maze of her emotions with the help of our team's counselling and psychology professionals. She was comforted by the acceptance of self-help and coping tactics, which strengthened her determination to break free from the limitations of her illness.

As her voyage progressed, an unexpected transformation started to occur inside of her. The tendrils of C. diff colitis, which had previously gripped her tightly, started to release their grasp. The threat of recurring infections subsided, making room for a renewed energy that resonated throughout her body. Through a journey that defied the usual course of her ailment, Mrs. Thompson's storey had come to represent the transformative power of holistic healthcare and wellbeing.

Her experience demonstrated the significant role that a complete lifestyle change may have in controlling and preventing C. diff colitis and provided hope for recovery and adaptability. A deep sense of inspiration and hope filled the audience as she wrapped up her storey, leaving a lasting impression on my mind. Mrs. Thompson's journey served as a tribute to the resilient spirit that each of us possessed, a spirit capable of overcoming adversity and setting out on a path to restored health and vitality.

In managing and preventing C. diff colitis, the storey of Mrs. Thompson's lifestyle makeover embodies the transformative power of holistic healthcare and wellbeing. Her storey shines a hope-filled light on a route that goes beyond the boundaries of traditional medical paradigms. Mrs. Thompson became a symbol of resiliency and rejuvenation by combining customised lifestyle adjustments, food planning, counselling and psychology-related methods, holistic therapies, self-care practises, and coping mechanisms.

Her experience demonstrates how the field of holistic health and wellness provides a tapestry of life-changing interventions with the potential to bring about restoration and vigour. It is an area where the fusion of complementary and evidence-based practises strengthens the human spirit and creates a haven of health that reaches beyond the confines of disease. Mrs. Thompson's storey entices us in, providing a window into the life-changing possibilities of a complete lifestyle makeover in the management and prevention of C. diff colitis—a possibility that speaks to everyone's desire for health and vitality.

Following Mrs. Thompson's storey, a deep realisation dawned, emphasising the critical role that dietary planning, lifestyle changes, and overall wellness play in managing and preventing C. diff colitis. Her experience is proof of the transformational power of adopting a multifaceted approach to wellness and health, one that offers the prospect of recovery and resiliency.

Her tale is a light of hope that points people—including medical professionals—in the direction of the life-changing potential of holistic healthcare and wellness as it echoes through the pages of medical literature. Through her journey, Mrs. Thompson provides us with a profound understanding of the tenacious spirit that each of us possesses—a spirit that can overcome adversity and steer toward a fresh sense of energy and wellbeing.

Mrs. Thompson's experience is a testimonial to the transformative power of a lifestyle overhaul in controlling and avoiding C. diff colitis in the field of holistic healthcare and wellness. Her storey ignites a torch of hope in the hearts of people facing the difficulties of disease by serving as an embodiment of resilience and rebirth. Her narrative calls us to a paradigm change toward a holistic strategy that supports a sanctuary of well-being and strengthens the resilience of the human spirit as it reverberates through the corridors of medical knowledge.

Medical Treatments and Approaches

Antibiotic Treatments

It is critical to comprehend the critical function that antibiotics play in treating C. difficile colitis as we dig into the intricate world of this condition's management. The use of antibiotics has been essential in the treatment of C. diff colitis; nevertheless, the rise in antibiotic resistance has presented a serious problem. We will go into great detail on the use of antibiotics in the treatment of C. diff colitis as well as any possible side effects related to resistance in this chapter. We will provide proof or anticipated results as we describe the main problems, emphasise the effects of antibiotic resistance, offer workable alternatives, and go into depth about how they should be implemented.

It is crucial to understand the historical background of antibiotic therapy in C. difficile colitis in order to set the stage for our discussion. Antibiotic use—clindamycin, fluoroquinolones, and cephalosporins in particular—has long been linked to the emergence of C. difficile infections. The alteration of the gut microbiota caused by the overuse and misuse of antibiotics has made it easier for C. difficile to colonise and infect people.

The main problem at hand is the increasing worry over the use of antibiotics in the management of C. difficile colitis. The effectiveness of standard antibiotics is reduced when C. difficile strains develop resistance to them, which can result in extended sickness, recurring infections, and higher healthcare expenses. The difficulty is in coming up with practical plans to fight antibiotic resistance and improve C. difficile colitis treatment.

The repercussions are severe if the issue of antibiotic resistance in C. difficile colitis is not sufficiently addressed. Extended sickness, repeated infections, and the risk of serious side effects like toxic megacolon and sepsis are all quite real. Furthermore, patients' and healthcare systems' financial burdens from extended hospital stays and the requirement for pricey alternative treatments would increase.

A diversified strategy to antibiotic treatment is essential given the urgent problem of antibiotic resistance. Promising approaches to managing antibiotic resistance in C. difficile colitis include the use of narrow-spectrum antibiotics, including fidaxomicin, and the investigation of complementary and alternative therapies, such as phage therapy and faecal microbiota transplantation (FMT).

A coordinated effort by researchers, politicians, and healthcare professionals is needed to put these proposals into practise. Strict antibiotic stewardship initiatives that maximise antibiotic utilisation, encourage prudent drug selection, and reduce needless exposure are crucial. Furthermore, standardised methods and continual research are required to validate the safety and efficacy of novel treatment modalities like phage therapy and FMT when integrating them into clinical practise.

The implementation of narrow-spectrum antibiotics and alternative therapeutic approaches has demonstrated encouraging results in reducing antibiotic resistance and enhancing the effectiveness of treatment for C. diff. colitis. Fidaxomicin administration has been shown in studies to improve patient outcomes and lower recurrence rates. In a similar vein, FMT has shown astounding promise in the fight against antibiotic resistance by eliminating C. difficile infection and diversifying the gut flora.

Although the remedies outlined above have great potential, it is important to recognise that there are other ways to address antibiotic resistance in C. difficile colitis. More investigation and assessment are needed into the creation of novel antimicrobial drugs that specifically target C. difficile, immunotherapeutic approaches, and the development of probiotics and prebiotics as supplemental therapies.

In conclusion, the problem of antibiotic resistance is closely related to the use of antibiotics in the treatment of C. diff. colitis. We can usher in a new era in the care of C. diff. colitis by thoroughly comprehending the seriousness of antibiotic resistance, putting forth complete remedies, and carefully carrying out these tactics. Together, researchers, politicians, and healthcare practitioners must fight antibiotic resistance and inaugurate in a new age of efficient and long-lasting C. diff. colitis treatment methods.

Surgical Options

As we delve more into the complex world of C. diff. colitis, it becomes clear that, in some situations, surgery becomes an essential part of managing this illness. The choice to seek surgical treatment for C. diff. colitis is frequently difficult and requires a thorough comprehension of the underlying causes, possible dangers, and expected results. We will explore the complexities of surgical treatments for C. diff. colitis in this chapter, explaining the indications, techniques, and aftercare to help clarify the role of surgery in managing this difficult condition.

Prior to discussing the particular surgical treatments for C. diff. colitis, it is necessary to clarify the signs and symptoms that warrant surgical intervention. Conservative approaches, including as antibiotic medication, supportive care, and, in certain circumstances, alternative therapeutic techniques like faecal microbiota transplantation, can be used to effectively control C. diff colitis in most patients. Surgical intervention becomes necessary, though, when the illness reaches a severe and refractory state that is marked by consequences including toxic megacolon, intestinal perforation, or persistent colitis that is not responding to medicinal therapy.

A variety of techniques are available for treating the consequences and underlying pathology of C. diff. colitis during surgery. These treatments can include more involved surgeries like a total colectomy with or without ileal pouch-anal anastomosis, or they can involve more limited resections of the afflicted bowel segments (IPAA). The degree of the illness, the patient's general condition, and the existence of complicating factors like immunosuppression or comorbidities all influence the surgical technique that is chosen.

Emergency surgery is crucial in cases of fulminant C. diff. colitis including a bowel perforation, whether it is imminent or already occurred. To minimise the danger of systemic sepsis and remove the infected colonic segments as soon as possible, a subtotal colectomy with end ileostomy may be necessary. On the other hand, a phased strategy might be taken into account for those whose colitis is not fullminant but is medically refractory. This may entail a diverting loop ileostomy in the beginning to relieve symptoms and facilitate colon healing, with bowel continuity being restored later.

Total proctocolectomy with end ileostomy or total colectomy with ileorectal anastomosis (IRA) may be considered in the setting of severe and recurrent C. diff colitis. But after an IRA, it is important to understand that the disease may return in the retained rectum, requiring close monitoring and possibly even another proctectomy if the condition worsens. To preserve bowel continuity and prevent a permanent stoma, IPAA can also be pursued in certain circumstances, especially in individuals with concurrent C. diff. colitis and ulcerative colitis.

The changing paradigms in the treatment of C. diff. colitis are reflected in the historical background of surgical options. Historically, surgery was mostly used for urgent cases involving a large colonic involvement, which frequently resulted in significant morbidity and the requirement for permanent ostomies. But thanks to developments in perioperative care, surgical methods, and the understanding of how C. diff. colitis affects quality of life, surgical management has changed to include a more customised and sophisticated approach.

The patient's clinical status, the severity of the disease, and the potential effects on long-term quality of life must all be taken into account while evaluating surgical alternatives for C. diff. colitis. Therefore, to ensure thorough patient evaluation, well-informed decision-making, and appropriate perioperative care, a multidisciplinary strategy combining gastroenterologists, colorectal surgeons, infectious disease specialists, and stoma care nurses is essential.

Consider the instance of a 45-year-old patient who has a history of recurrent C. diff. colitis that is not responsive to antibiotic therapy in order to demonstrate the use of surgical options in the setting of C. diff. colitis. The patient still has debilitating symptoms and recurrent episodes of colitis despite receiving numerous rounds of conventional and alternative treatments, such as fidaxomicin and faecal microbiota transplantation. The interdisciplinary team in this case decides that surgery is necessary and proceeds with a total colectomy and IPAA, giving the patient a long-lasting and effective outcome in the end.

Common Misconceptions or Misinterpretations

One common misperception regarding surgical treatments for C. diff. colitis is that surgery is a last resort or a sign that medicinal care has failed. Surgery is, in fact, an essential supplement to the overall therapy of C. diff. colitis, providing the chance to resolve the illness, enhance quality of life, and prevent the recurrence of incapacitating chronic symptoms.

Finally, taking into account surgical options for the treatment of C. diff. colitis is an essential part of an all-encompassing strategy for managing this difficult condition. We want to give patients, their families, and healthcare professionals a complete grasp of how surgery can treat C. diff. colitis by clarifying the indications, protocols, and postoperative issues related to surgical interventions. We can successfully traverse the challenges of surgical management and work to improve patient outcomes in the treatment of this condition by working together and making well-informed decisions.

Fecal Microbiota Transplantation (FMT)

The therapy of C. diff. colitis is frequently complex, necessitating a thorough knowledge of several approaches to treatment. Fecal microbiota transplantation (FMT), which offers a novel therapeutic method targeted at reestablishing the balance of the gut microbiota, has emerged as a viable treatment for recurrent and refractory C. difficile colitis. This chapter will clarify the nuances of this novel treatment approach by examining the idea of FMT, its success rate, and the requirements for possible candidacy.

Fecal material from a healthy donor is sent into the gastrointestinal tract of a recipient in a process called faecal bacteriotherapy, or FMT for short. The aim of this treatment is to help the recipient's gut repopulate with a varied and healthy microbial community. By taking advantage of the symbiotic interaction between the gut microbiota and host health, this procedure can potentially resolve dysbiosis and restore microbiota, which is a defining feature of C. difficile colitis. A wide range of commensal bacteria, viruses, fungi, and metabolites are present in the transplanted faecal material, which comes from carefully chosen donors. These microorganisms work together to support the recovery of microbial diversity and function in the recipient's gut environment.

A notable example of the efficacy of FMT in the management of C. Diff. Colitis is exemplified by a 55-year-old patient with a history of recurrent and refractory C. Diff. Colitis unresponsive to conventional antibiotic therapy. Following the administration of FMT, obtained from a thoroughly screened and healthy donor, the patient experienced a rapid resolution of symptoms and a sustained remission of the disease. This case underscores the potential for FMT to serve as a transformative intervention in the context of C. Diff. Colitis, offering a curative solution for individuals burdened by the challenges of recurrent and refractory disease.

Despite the fact that FMT has shown to be remarkably effective in treating C. diff. colitis, it is important to recognise the various viewpoints that surround this therapeutic approach. Regarding the treatment of recurrent and refractory C. diff colitis, FMT is a revolutionary approach that offers a rare chance to address the underlying dysbiosis and reestablish gut homeostasis. However, a sophisticated approach to the wider application of FMT is required because to ethical considerations, regulatory frameworks, and logistical challenges around donor screening and material processing. Furthermore, research projects are being carried out to clarify the long-term safety, effectiveness, and possible uses of FMT outside of C. diff colitis, which will contribute to the conversation about this novel treatment modality.

There is strong evidence to support the effectiveness of FMT when it comes to managing recurrent and refractory C. difficile colitis, as demonstrated by an examination of its success rates. Research has indicated that after a single FMT surgery, resolution rates can reach over 85%, and most responding patients experience persistent remission. Moreover, the comparative efficacy of FMT exceeds that of traditional antibiotic therapy, highlighting the intervention's transformative potential in the setting of C. difficile colitis. These results validate the efficacy of FMT as a first-line treatment option for patients coping with recurrent and resistant illness.

A dysbiosis is defined as an imbalance or disruption in the gut microbiota's composition and function, marked by a proinflammatory microbial milieu, a decrease in microbial diversity, and an altered community structure. One of the main characteristics of C. difficile colitis is dysbiosis, which plays a role in both the disease's pathophysiology and the duration of recurring symptoms. By restoring microbial diversity and functionality, FMT seeks to reduce dysbiosis and foster a healthy gut ecology that is beneficial to the host's well-being.

Finally, FMT offers a strong therapeutic option for microbial restoration and illness resolution, making it a crucial tool in the treatment of recurrent and resistant C. difficile colitis. The significance of FMT in the management of C. diff. colitis is highlighted by its success rates and its ability to change the clinical trajectory of persons facing recurrent illness difficulties. FMT is a treatment option for people struggling with the intricacies of recurrent and refractory C. difficile colitis, and it provides hope within the constantly changing landscape of therapeutic methods.

Alternative Medicine and C. Diff

Recent years have seen a considerable increase in interest in the application of alternative medicine to the treatment of C. diff. colitis, with proponents arguing that these approaches may be effective in tackling the difficulties this complicated condition presents. In order to give a thorough grasp of alternative medicine modalities' place in the therapeutic landscape, it is crucial to critically assess the claims and evidence surrounding them as C. diff. colitis therapy continues to change.

The main argument being investigated is the effectiveness of complementary and alternative medicine techniques in treating C. diff. colitis symptoms and recurrence, with an emphasis on how well they can balance the gut microbiota and treat dysbiosis.

The use of probiotics is one of the main complementary and alternative medicine methods that has gained interest in relation to C. difficile colitis. Probiotics have been proposed as a possible adjuvant therapy to standard antibiotic treatment in addressing the dysbiosis associated with C. difficile colitis. Probiotics are defined as live microorganisms that give health benefits to the host when administered in suitable doses. Research has indicated that some probiotic strains, specifically those from the Lactobacillus and Bifidobacterium genera, may have positive impacts on gut barrier function and microbial diversity restoration, which may help alleviate the symptoms of C. diff. colitis.

It is hypothesised that probiotics' capacity to alter the composition and function of the gut microbiota is how they might have a positive impact on C. difficile colitis. Probiotics may inhibit the growth of pathogenic Clostridioides difficile and lessen its virulence by competing with the pathogen for adherence sites and nutrients in the gut. This could potentially lower the risk of C. difficile colitis development and recurrence. Additionally, it has been demonstrated that some probiotic strains increase mucosal barrier integrity and induce the synthesis of antimicrobial peptides, which may have protective effects against C. difficile colonisation and infection.

Although probiotics hold theoretical potential for mitigating dysbiosis and C. difficile-associated diseases, there is divergent evidence and opinion regarding their effectiveness when it comes to C. difficile colitis. There are concerns regarding the robustness of probiotics as a stand-alone or supplementary treatment intervention because some studies have found minimal or equivocal benefits of probiotics in preventing C. difficile infection or reducing its recurrence. Furthermore, the variability observed in the probiotic strains, doses, and formulations employed in clinical trials poses challenges to the interpretation of their overall effectiveness and their applicability to a wider range of persons afflicted with C. difficile colitis.

It is crucial to acknowledge the difficulties in determining the effectiveness of probiotics in the setting of C. diff. colitis in light of the counter-evidence. It's possible that variations in C. difficile strains, patient groups, and study designs are to blame for the inconsistent results reported in the literature. Furthermore, in the setting of C. diff. colitis, customised methods to probiotic therapy are necessary due to the interaction between probiotic formulations and host variables, including the immune system and the composition of the gut microbiota at present. Despite the limitations and contradicting evidence, more research efforts are necessary to identify the precise circumstances in which probiotics may provide the best advantages in the treatment of C. diff. colitis.

Apart from probiotics, the potential role of alternative medicine methods such herbal medicines and traditional Chinese medicine in treating C. diff. colitis has been investigated. In preclinical trials, certain herbal formulations, such berberine and curcumin, have demonstrated antibacterial and anti-inflammatory activities; this suggests a possible direction for further research in the context of managing C. diff. colitis. Proponents of traditional Chinese medicine have suggested using acupuncture and herbal formulations as supplemental therapies to traditional treatment plans. They claim that these approaches can regulate immune responses and help restore gut homeostasis.

In conclusion, investigating alternative medicine treatments in the context of C. diff. colitis reveals a landscape with a variety of claims and supporting data, requiring a careful and evidence-based assessment process. Probiotics and some herbal therapies may be able to help with dysbiosis and modify host-microbiota interactions, but more thorough clinical research and individualised treatment plans are still required. The intricate interactions among host variables, alternative medicine modalities, and the pathophysiology of C. difficile colitis highlight the need for ongoing research to define their possible significance in the all-encompassing treatment of this difficult illness. In the context of C. diff. colitis, navigating the complexities of alternative medicine requires a careful, evidence-based approach to fully understand their therapeutic potential.

Immunotherapy and Future Treatments

With the advent of immunotherapy and its potential to revolutionise the treatment of this complicated ailment, the field of C. diff. colitis therapeutic treatments has seen tremendous strides in recent years. Immunotherapy, a therapeutic approach that utilises the body's immune system to fight illnesses, has drawn interest due to its potential to alleviate the problems caused by colitis and C. difficile infection. This chapter explores the development of immunotherapy in relation to C. diff. colitis, outlining significant turning points, talking about contemporary interpretations and modifications, and addressing issues and disputes that have influenced the course of the treatment.

The earliest known instances of immunotherapy date from the late 1800s, when surgeon William Coley noticed that certain cancer patients' tumours shrank as a result of bacterial infections. This coincidental finding established the basis for the theory of using the immune system to fight illness, which is when immunotherapy first emerged. The investigation of immunotherapy in the context of infectious disorders, such as C. diff. colitis, began as a result of Coley's observations, which generated interest in the potential of immunostimulatory drugs to treat a variety of ailments.

1. Early Immunomodulatory Agents: An important turning point in the development of immunotherapy was the introduction of early immunomodulatory drugs like interleukins and interferons. These agents were originally investigated for their potential to treat infectious diseases, such as those caused by C. difficile. However, they also provided insights into the complex interactions between the immune system and disease pathogenesis, laying the foundation for future research into these agents' potential applications.

2. Monoclonal Antibodies: Targeted immunotherapy underwent a radical transformation with the introduction of monoclonal antibodies. Monoclonal antibodies provided a customised method of

battling diseases because of their ability to precisely target and eliminate disease-causing pathogens. Monoclonal antibodies that target C. difficile toxins and surface antigens have emerged as a potentially effective therapy option for C. difficile colitis, with the ability to reduce the severity and recurrence of the disease.

3. Fecal Microbiota Transplantation (FMT): FMT is a novel treatment strategy that restores gut microbial diversity to control the host's immune response, even though it is not traditionally classified as immunotherapy. The gut microbiota-immune axis plays a critical role in the management of disease, as evidenced by the exceptional success of FMT, which transfers healthy donor faecal microbiota to a recipient, in treating recurrent C. diff. colitis.

Diagrams that illustrate the mechanisms of action of immunotherapeutic drugs, such as FMT and monoclonal antibodies, can be used as visual aids to improve comprehension of these intricate treatment methods. Furthermore, readers can gain important insights from histopathological images that show the immunopathology of C. diff. colitis and the possible influence of immunotherapy on disease pathology.

In the setting of C. diff. colitis, immunotherapy has developed against a background of regional and cultural differences in treatment modalities and patient preferences. While some areas have accepted immunotherapy as the mainstay of managing C. difficile infections, others have taken a more cautious stance, highlighting the necessity of culturally aware and customised interventions to address the various ways that C. difficile colitis manifests itself in various populations.

In the context of C. difficile colitis, contemporary interpretations of immunotherapy include a range of cutting-edge strategies, such as the creation of novel immunomodulatory drugs that target certain immunological pathways linked to the pathophysiology of C. difficile. Moreover, the amalgamation of immunomodulatory tactics with traditional antibiotic treatment and the investigation of customised immunotherapeutic regimens highlight the ever-changing terrain of contemporary immunotherapy modifications in managing the intricacies of C. difficile colitis management.

Immunotherapy's voyage in the field of C. difficile colitis has been dotted with significant obstacles and disputes, the most significant of which being the possibility of immunosuppression and immune response dysregulation in the context of C. difficile infection. The intricate equilibrium between augmenting immune-mediated elimination of C. difficile and averting immunopathology presents a noteworthy obstacle in the development and execution of immunotherapeutic approaches. Furthermore, there are debates concerning the long-term safety and effectiveness of immunomodulatory drugs in the setting of C. diff. colitis, which makes a careful analysis of the advantages and disadvantages of these treatments necessary.

The addition of immunotherapy to the C. diff. colitis treatment regimen signifies a paradigm change in the strategy for managing this difficult illness. Through the complex interactions between the immune system, gut microbiota, and the pathogenesis of C. difficile, immunotherapy may provide customised immune-focused treatments to supplement conventional antibiotic regimens and address the complex nature of C. difficile colitis.

Anticipating the future, novel immunotherapeutic approaches such as immune checkpoint inhibitors, microbiota-targeted immunomodulators, and genetically modified immune cells are expected to revolutionise immunotherapy in the setting of C. diff. colitis. These innovative methods seek to take use of the growing body of knowledge regarding the relationships between the host, microbiota, and immune system and open the door for precision immunotherapy in the treatment of colitis brought on by C. difficile infection.

Conclusion

To sum up, the development of immunotherapy in the context of C. diff. colitis is a path characterised by pivotal moments, continuous adjustments, and the possibility of customised immune-focused therapies. In order to effectively address the difficulties caused by C. difficile infection, we must critically assess immunotherapy as we work to identify the best approaches that balance immunological risk reduction with maximal therapeutic efficacy. Immunotherapy has a bright future in the context of C. difficile colitis; it will usher in a new era of immune-centric, tailored treatments that try to simplify the complex workings of this complex illness.

Navigating Treatment Options

Both patients and healthcare professionals face substantial challenges when managing C. difficile colitis. The need for efficient treatment alternatives has increased due to the rise in antibiotic resistance and recurrent illnesses. Patients must be able to make educated decisions about their care by having a thorough understanding of the intricacies of this ailment and the range of treatment options available. This chapter will examine the present state of C. difficile colitis treatment choices and offer insights into the decision-making process.

The bacteria Clostridium difficile is the source of C. difficile colitis, a serious and potentially fatal colon infection. The main problem is that C. difficile can create toxins that harm the colon's lining, causing symptoms that can range from moderate diarrhoea to severe inflammation and colonic perforation. The high recurrence rates of this illness and the poor effectiveness of traditional antibiotic therapies provide management challenges.

C. difficile colitis can lead to longer hospital stays, higher medical expenses, and in extreme situations, death if treatment is not received. Recurrent infections have a substantial emotional and financial toll in addition to having an adverse effect on the patient's physical condition. The therapy of C. difficile colitis is further complicated by the overuse of antibiotics, which adds to the growing concern about antibiotic resistance.

Given the difficulties associated with C. difficile colitis, it is critical to investigate alternate therapy modalities that tackle the drawbacks of conventional antibiotic treatments. Fecal microbiota transplantation (FMT), a novel strategy for reestablishing the equilibrium of the gut microbiota and getting rid of C. difficile infection, is one such promising treatment. In order to restore a varied and healthy microbiome in the recipient's gastrointestinal tract, FMT entails transferring faecal material from a healthy donor.

First, a qualified donor must be chosen, and then there are various important actions to take in order to confirm that no potential pathogens are present. Strict protocols must be followed during the collection, processing, and administration of faecal material in order to reduce the possibility of unfavourable outcomes. Whether a colonoscopy, nasogastric tube, or oral capsules are used, the administration method should be customised for each patient according to their preferences and clinical status. It is imperative to closely observe the patient following transplantation in order to evaluate the procedure's efficacy and safety.

Numerous studies have demonstrated high rates of remission and a considerable reduction in the risk of recurrence, confirming the efficacy of FMT in the treatment of recurrent C. difficile infection. By lowering the dependency on antimicrobial medications, the restoration of a healthy gut microbiome via FMT not only addresses the fundamental cause of C. difficile colitis but also presents a viable defence against antibiotic resistance.

Even though FMT has been remarkably effective in treating C. difficile colitis, it is important to recognise that there are other treatment options available. These could include the creation of vaccinations to guard against C. difficile infection, innovative antimicrobial drugs with limited spectrum activity, and experimental treatments such monoclonal antibodies that target C. difficile toxins. Adding further therapy choices to the arsenal for C. difficile colitis requires assessing these substitutes in light of their long-term effects, safety, and effectiveness.

In summary, the field of C. difficile colitis treatment options is changing and offering patients a variety of options that were not previously available. Achieving success in managing C. difficile colitis requires navigating the complicated topography of treatment modalities, assessing potential benefits and risks, and participating in collaborative decision-making with healthcare providers. Patients can empower themselves to make decisions that are in line with their unique requirements and preferences by adopting cutting-edge technologies like FMT and actively engaging in the decision-making process.Both patients and healthcare professionals face substantial challenges when managing C. difficile colitis. The need for efficient treatment alternatives has increased due to the rise in antibiotic resistance and recurrent illnesses. Patients must be able to make educated decisions about their care by having a thorough understanding of the intricacies of this ailment and the range of treatment options available. This chapter will examine the present state of C. difficile colitis treatment choices and offer insights into the decision-making process.

The bacteria Clostridium difficile is the source of C. difficile colitis, a serious and potentially fatal colon infection. The main problem is that C. difficile can create toxins that harm the colon's lining, causing symptoms that can range from moderate diarrhoea to severe inflammation and colonic perforation. The high recurrence rates of this illness and the poor effectiveness of traditional antibiotic therapies provide management challenges.

C. difficile colitis can lead to longer hospital stays, higher medical expenses, and in extreme situations, death if treatment is not received. Recurrent infections have a substantial emotional and financial toll in addition to having an adverse effect on the patient's physical condition. The therapy of C. difficile colitis is further complicated by the overuse of antibiotics, which adds to the growing concern about antibiotic resistance.

Given the difficulties associated with C. difficile colitis, it is critical to investigate alternate therapy modalities that tackle the drawbacks of conventional antibiotic treatments. Fecal microbiota transplantation (FMT), a novel strategy for reestablishing the equilibrium of the gut microbiota and getting rid of C. difficile infection, is one such promising treatment. In order to restore a varied and healthy microbiome in the recipient's gastrointestinal tract, FMT entails transferring faecal material from a healthy donor.

First, a qualified donor must be chosen, and then there are various important actions to take in order to confirm that no potential pathogens are present. Strict protocols must be followed during the collection, processing, and administration of faecal material in order to reduce the possibility of unfavourable outcomes. Whether a colonoscopy, nasogastric tube, or oral capsules are used, the administration method should be customised for each patient according to their preferences and clinical status. It is imperative to closely observe the patient following transplantation in order to evaluate the procedure's efficacy and safety.

Numerous studies have demonstrated high rates of remission and a considerable reduction in the risk of recurrence, confirming the efficacy of FMT in the treatment of recurrent C. difficile infection. By lowering the dependency on antimicrobial medications, the restoration of a healthy gut microbiome via FMT not only addresses the fundamental cause of C. difficile colitis but also presents a viable defence against antibiotic resistance.

Even though FMT has been remarkably effective in treating C. difficile colitis, it is important to recognise that there are other treatment options available. These could include the creation of vaccinations to guard against C. difficile infection, innovative antimicrobial drugs with limited spectrum activity, and experimental treatments such monoclonal antibodies that target C. difficile toxins. Adding further therapy choices to the arsenal for C. difficile colitis requires assessing these substitutes in light of their long-term effects, safety, and effectiveness.

In summary, the field of C. difficile colitis treatment options is changing and offering patients a variety of options that were not previously available. Achieving success in managing C. difficile colitis requires navigating the complicated topography of treatment modalities, assessing potential benefits and risks, and participating in collaborative decision-making with healthcare providers. Patients can empower themselves to make decisions that are in line with their unique requirements and preferences by adopting cutting-edge technologies like FMT and actively engaging in the decision-making process.

Coping With C. Diff. Colitis

Coping Mechanisms for Chronic Illness

There are many obstacles to overcome when dealing with a chronic condition, like C. diff. colitis, which calls for useful coping mechanisms. The essential coping strategies that have been demonstrated to be helpful for people managing the difficulties of chronic diseases are outlined in the list below. These systems are designed to give people dealing with the day-to-day effects of these illnesses courage, support, and a sense of empowerment. Through comprehension and application of these tactics, people can develop an increased sense of authority over their physical and mental welfare.

a. The capacity to identify, comprehend, and efficiently control one's emotions in reaction to the difficulties presented by a chronic illness is referred to as emotional regulation. It entails developing flexible coping mechanisms to manage the mental turmoil that frequently accompanies persistent health issues. Anxiety, frustration, and dread are just a few of the feelings that people with C. diff. colitis may have. These feelings can have a very negative influence on their quality of life. People can lessen the negative consequences of these emotions and promote a more stable and resilient psychological state by learning emotional control strategies.

Psychology research has emphasised the significance of emotional regulation in fostering psychological health, especially when chronic illness is involved. Research has indicated that those with strong emotional regulation abilities display reduced levels of discomfort and higher levels of adaptive functioning when faced with health-related obstacles. Moreover, testimonies from people with long-term illnesses emphasise the game-changing effect that emotional regulation techniques have on improving their capacity to manage the day-to-day challenges associated with their sickness.

Cognitive-behavioral treatments like cognitive restructuring and thought challenging are examples of practical applications of emotional regulation strategies that help people reframe negative thinking patterns and develop more adaptive attitudes about their illness. Furthermore, mindfulness-based techniques like progressive muscle relaxation and deep breathing exercises can be extremely helpful in reducing emotional discomfort and fostering serenity in the midst of the chaos that comes with a chronic illness. People can improve their overall well-being by proactively addressing the emotional upheaval associated with C. diff. colitis by implementing these useful applications into their daily lives.

After discussing the fundamental significance of emotional regulation, we now focus on the critical function that social support plays in promoting resilience and coping effectiveness for those who are dealing with chronic disease.

a. The network of personal connections and resources that people can rely on to get informational, practical, and emotional help in times of need is referred to as social support. Social support is crucial for mitigating the negative effects of C. diff. colitis and promoting a feeling of community and connection among individuals coping with its challenges. A strong social support system, whether it comes from friends, family, medical professionals, or support groups, can greatly lessen the stress of a chronic illness and improve coping skills in general.

Research continuously highlights the positive impacts of social support on health outcomes, especially when it comes to managing chronic illnesses. Research has indicated that those who possess robust social support networks tend to exhibit reduced levels of psychological distress, better quality of life, and increased adherence to treatment. Furthermore, personal testimonies from people managing C. diff. colitis confirm the critical function of social support in offering consolation, comprehension, and useful help during the trying path of chronic illness.

In order to effectively use social support, one must deliberately seek out and cultivate genuine relationships that provide comprehension, empathy, and practical help. This could mean speaking candidly and openly with loved ones about one's needs and difficulties, attending support groups designed especially for people with C. diff. colitis, and using community resources to get pertinent information and services. People can strengthen their coping mechanisms and develop a sense of resilience in the face of the complex demands posed by chronic disease by utilising the power of social support.

Now that we have a thorough grasp of the critical role that social support plays, we can move on to discuss the importance of self-care and lifestyle changes as vital coping strategies for people navigating the challenges of chronic illnesses like C. diff. colitis.

Mental Health and Emotional Well-being

Managing Crohn's disease (C. diff. colitis) is a complex issue that affects a person's mental and emotional state in addition to their physical symptoms. Living with a chronic condition, like C. diff. colitis, can have significant psychological impacts, making a complete approach to emotional health maintenance necessary.

The principal concern under consideration is the psychological cost associated with the management of C. diff. colitis, encompassing worry, despair, dread, and uncertainty, among other things. The illness's unpredictable character, the physical suffering it brings, and the disruption it causes to daily life can all lead to these emotional difficulties.

Ignoring the psychological effects of C. diff. colitis can have a number of negative effects, such as worsening physical symptoms, lowering quality of life, causing interpersonal conflicts, and reducing treatment compliance. Additionally, the emotional load may exacerbate a distressing cycle that impedes general wellbeing and efficient coping.

Integrating evidence-based techniques that support psychological resilience, encourage adaptive coping, and foster a positive outlook in the face of persistent health issues is a holistic approach to preserving emotional health.

Incorporating mindfulness-based practises into everyday routines, actively seeking out social support to promote a sense of connection and understanding, and attending psychotherapy to address specific emotional concerns are some practical steps that can be taken to put emotional well-being strategies into practise.

The benefits of treating the psychological impacts of chronic illness on general well-being have been shown by research. People who take proactive measures to preserve their emotional well-being may see improvements in their quality of life, decreased psychological discomfort, and increased coping efficacy.

Although the suggested remedies are sound, it's also critical to recognise that there are other strategies that can improve mental wellbeing for people with C. diff. colitis. These strategies include expressive writing interventions, peer support groups, and creative therapies.

Beyond its physical manifestations, C. diff. colitis can pose serious obstacles to daily living. Managing with chronic condition can have a significant emotional toll, making a thorough strategy for preserving mental health and emotional well-being necessary. The psychological effects of C. diff. colitis will be discussed in detail in the parts that follow, along with evidence-based methods for enhancing emotional health and helpful hints for incorporating these methods into day-to-day activities.

Living with C. diff. colitis can have severe psychological repercussions, including a variety of emotional difficulties that have a substantial negative influence on an individual's quality of life. It is crucial to recognise and manage the psychological effects of this long-term illness in order to build resilience and enhance general quality of life.

The main concern here is the psychological cost of treating C. diff. colitis, which can present as worry, uncertainty, anxiety, and sadness. These psychological difficulties may result from the disease's unpredictable nature, the suffering it brings about physically, and the interruption it causes to day-to-day activities.

Neglecting to tackle the psychological effects of Crohn's disease can result in unfavourable consequences such as heightened physical symptoms, damaged social bonds, less treatment compliance, and compromised general health. Emotional anguish can create a vicious cycle that makes it difficult to cope and jeopardises mental health.

Integrating evidence-based techniques that support psychological resilience, encourage adaptive coping, and foster a positive outlook in the face of persistent health issues is a holistic approach to preserving emotional health.

Incorporating mindfulness-based practises into everyday routines, actively seeking out social support to promote a sense of connection and understanding, and attending psychotherapy to address specific emotional concerns are some practical steps that can be taken to put emotional well-being strategies into practise.

The benefits of treating the psychological impacts of chronic illness on general well-being have been shown by research. People who take proactive measures to preserve their emotional well-being may see improvements in their quality of life, decreased psychological discomfort, and increased coping efficacy.

Although the suggested remedies are sound, it's also critical to recognise that there are other strategies that can improve mental wellbeing for people with C. diff. colitis. These strategies include expressive writing interventions, peer support groups, and creative therapies.

Understanding the Psychological Impact of C. Diff. Colitis

C. Diff. Colitis, as a chronic illness, presents a myriad of challenges that extend beyond the physical symptoms it entails. In navigating the complexities of this condition, individuals often encounter profound psychological effects that can significantly influence their emotional well-being. It is imperative to recognize the psychological toll of managing C. Diff. Colitis and to develop effective strategies to maintain mental health and emotional well-being in the face of these challenges.

The psychological effects of living with C. Diff. Colitis can be profound, encompassing a range of emotional challenges that significantly impact an individual's well-being. Understanding and addressing the psychological toll of this chronic illness is essential for fostering resilience and promoting overall quality of life.

The primary issue at hand pertains to the psychological burden of managing C. Diff. Colitis, which may manifest as anxiety, depression, fear, and uncertainty. These emotional challenges can arise from the unpredictability of the illness, the physical discomfort it causes, and the disruption it imposes on daily life.

Failing to address the psychological impact of C. Diff. Colitis can lead to adverse outcomes, including exacerbation of physical symptoms, strained interpersonal relationships, decreased treatment adherence, and impaired overall well-being. The emotional burden can perpetuate a cycle of distress that hinders effective coping and compromises mental health.

A comprehensive approach to maintaining emotional health involves integrating evidence-based strategies that bolster psychological resilience, promote adaptive coping, and cultivate a positive outlook in the face of ongoing health challenges.

Practical steps to implement emotional well-being strategies may include engaging in psychotherapy to address specific emotional concerns, integrating mindfulness-based practices into daily routines, and actively seeking out social support to foster a sense of connectedness and understanding.

Research has demonstrated the positive impact of addressing the psychological effects of chronic illness on overall well-being. By adopting proactive strategies to maintain emotional health, individuals may experience reduced psychological distress, enhanced coping efficacy, and improved quality of life.

While the proposed solutions are foundational, it is also important to acknowledge alternative approaches, such as peer support groups, expressive writing interventions, and creative therapies, which may complement and enhance emotional well-being for individuals managing C. Diff. Colitis.

Understanding the Psychological Impact of C. Diff. Colitis

C. Diff. Colitis, being a chronic condition, poses numerous difficulties that go beyond its outward manifestations. People frequently experience deep psychological impacts while negotiating the complexities of this condition, which can have a substantial impact on their emotional well-being. It's critical to acknowledge the psychological costs associated with controlling C. diff. colitis and to create practical plans for preserving mental and emotional stability in the face of these difficulties.

Managing Crohn's disease (C. diff. colitis) is a complex issue that affects a person's mental and emotional state in addition to their physical symptoms. Living with a chronic condition, like C. diff. colitis, can have significant psychological impacts, making a complete approach to emotional health maintenance necessary.

Outline the primary issue or challenge in clear terms.

Detail what could happen if the problem is not addressed.

Propose a method or strategy to solve the identified issue.

Explain the steps to put the solution into action.

Provide evidence or projections of the solution's efficacy.

Mention and evaluate other possible solutions.

Living with C. diff. colitis can have severe psychological repercussions, including a variety of emotional difficulties that have a substantial negative influence on an individual's quality of life. It is crucial to recognise and manage the psychological effects of this long-term illness in order to build resilience and enhance general quality of life.

Managing Crohn's disease (C. diff. colitis) is a complex issue that affects a person's mental and emotional state in addition to their physical symptoms. Living with a chronic condition, like C. diff. colitis, can have significant psychological impacts, making a complete approach to emotional health maintenance necessary.

The main concern here is the psychological cost of treating C. diff. colitis, which can present as worry, uncertainty, anxiety, and sadness. These psychological difficulties may result from the disease's unpredictable nature, the suffering it brings about physically, and the interruption it causes to day-to-day activities.

Neglecting to tackle the psychological effects of Crohn's disease can result in unfavourable consequences such as heightened physical symptoms, damaged social bonds, less treatment compliance, and compromised general health. Emotional anguish can create a vicious cycle that makes it difficult to cope and jeopardises mental health.

Building Resilience

This section aims to provide people with techniques for building psychological toughness when dealing with C. diff. colitis. By offering readers a thorough road map for building resilience, the book will help them manage the emotional complexities of living with a chronic illness and improve their general well-being.

Readers will benefit from an open mentality, a desire to engage in introspection, and a dedication to incorporating the recommended tactics into their daily lives in order to accomplish the aim of building resilience. Furthermore, the process of building resilience can be made even more effective by having access to peer support groups, mental health specialists, and mindfulness tools.

In order to manage C. diff. colitis, building resilience requires a multimodal strategy that includes behavioural, emotional, and psychological techniques. To handle the challenges of chronic illness with greater adaptability and strength, this process involves acknowledging and addressing the psychological burden of the condition, incorporating evidence-based coping strategies, and cultivating a positive mentality.

The first steps in constructing resilience are self-awareness and comprehension of the particular psychological difficulties involved with controlling C. diff. colitis. To improve emotional well-being, this entails recognising and managing emotions, developing flexible coping strategies, creating social support systems, and including mindfulness exercises. Every stage contributes to a comprehensive strategy for emotional health and is closely related to the main objective of resilience-building.

It is crucial that people approach the process of developing resilience with self-compassion and tolerance as they set out on their path. Recognize that developing resilience is a slow and continuous process, and that experiencing setbacks or times of increased emotional vulnerabiity is normal. Practicing self-care, getting help from professionals when necessary, and keeping up a support system can all offer helpful tools and direction during this life-changing journey.

Increased psychological flexibility, better adaptive coping mechanisms, higher emotional regulation, and a stronger sense of empowerment in overcoming the difficulties of managing C. diff. colitis are indicators that the resilience-building process has been completed successfully. By considering their emotional reactions, behavioural patterns, and general sense of well-being in relation to managing their chronic illness, people can evaluate their success.

Building Resilience in the Context of C. Diff. Colitis

C. Diff. Colitis poses serious psychological and emotional obstacles in addition to physical difficulties. Maintaining emotional well-being in the face of chronic illness necessitates a planned and all-encompassing strategy to resilience development. The goal of this part is to give readers a road map for developing psychological resilience, giving them the skills and knowledge needed to successfully negotiate the challenges of controlling C. diff. colitis.

In order to manage C. diff. colitis, the goal of this section is to walk people through the process of building psychological resilience. Readers will learn how to build resilience and improve emotional well-being by following this step-by-step action and strategy guide.

People who are prepared to reflect on themselves, have an open mind, and have access to peer support groups and mental health specialists will find it easier to start the process of developing resilience. Furthermore, the successful development of resilience requires a dedication to putting the recommended techniques and practises into practise.

In the context of controlling C. diff. colitis, resilience building entails a multimodal strategy that includes psychological awareness, adaptive coping mechanisms, and the development of an optimistic outlook. Through this process, people will be able to manage the particular emotional difficulties that come with having a chronic illness and will be more equipped to handle their emotional ups and downs.

The first step towards developing resilience is realising the psychological effects of C. diff. colitis. To support individuals in managing the emotional complexities of chronic illness, this involves integrating mindfulness practises into daily routines, fostering social support networks, developing adaptive coping mechanisms, and recognising and processing emotions. All of these steps contribute to the overall goal of resilience-building.

It's critical to approach the process of developing resilience with self-compassion and tolerance as people embark on it. Understand that developing resilience is a gradual process, and that obstacles are normal to face along the road. During this process of transformation, seeking expert counsel, practising self-care, and keeping up a support system can offer invaluable resources and assistance.

Increased psychological flexibility, better coping mechanisms, higher emotional regulation, and a stronger sense of empowerment in handling the difficulties of C. diff. colitis are indicators that the resilience-building process has been completed successfully. By considering their emotional reactions, behavioural patterns, and general sense of well-being in relation to managing their chronic illness, people can evaluate their success.

Developing Psychological Resilience in the Context of C. Diff. Colitis

C. Diff. Colitis is a complex challenge to individuals that goes beyond physical symptoms and has a considerable psychological and emotional impact. A crucial part of preserving general wellbeing is the process of building psychological resilience in the face of chronic illness. The goal of this part is to give readers a thorough road map for developing resilience, giving them the tools they need to successfully manage C. diff. colitis.

This section aims to provide guidance to individuals on how to build psychological resilience within the framework of controlling C. diff. colitis in an organised manner. Through the provision of a step-by-step action plan and methods, readers will gain the necessary tools to cultivate resilience and improve their mental health.

People who are prepared to reflect on themselves, have an open mind, and have access to peer support groups and mental health specialists will find it easier to start the process of developing resilience. A dedication to putting the recommended methods and tactics into practise is also essential for the successful development of resilience.

When it comes to managing C. diff. colitis, building resilience is a comprehensive strategy that incorporates psychological awareness, adaptable coping mechanisms, and the development of an optimistic outlook. By addressing the particular emotional difficulties brought on by long-term sickness, this all-encompassing approach seeks to enable people to go through their health journeys with resilience and fortitude.

The first step towards developing resilience is realising the psychological effects of C. diff. colitis. This entails identifying and managing emotions, developing flexible coping strategies, building social support systems, and incorporating mindfulness exercises into regular activities. Every phase advances the overall objective of resilience-building, providing people with a thorough method for handling the psychological challenges of long-term illness.

It is crucial that people approach the process of developing resilience with self-compassion and tolerance as they set out on their path. Understand that developing resilience is a slow and continuous process, and that obstacles are normal to face along the road. During this process of transformation, seeking expert counsel, practising self-care, and keeping up a support system can offer invaluable resources and assistance.

Increased psychological flexibility, better coping mechanisms, higher emotional regulation, and a stronger sense of empowerment in handling the difficulties of C. diff. colitis are indicators that the resilience-building process has been completed successfully. By considering their emotional reactions, behavioural patterns, and general sense of well-being in relation to managing their chronic illness, people can evaluate their success.

I've carried on the book by exploring how to develop resilience when dealing with C. diff. colitis. I have concentrated on giving readers a thorough implementation roadmap, stressing the significance of each phase and providing direction for a smooth transition. Tell me if you want me to go on or if there's anything in particular you'd like me to concentrate on.

Support Groups and Community Resources

The advantages of attending support groups and making use of local resources become more and more clear as people work through the difficulties associated with controlling C. diff. colitis. The purpose of this section is to provide people with C. diff. colitis with an overview of the value of support systems and community services, including their possible effects on mental health, managing the condition, and general quality of life.

The management of C. diff. colitis include not only the medical therapies and physical symptoms but also the significant emotional and psychological effects that come with having a chronic condition. Understanding the complicated nature of the problems that patients encounter and the vital role that community services and support organisations play in helping to resolve these issues requires an appreciation of their diversity.

The main problem at hand is the emotional strain and sense of loneliness that people with C. diff. colitis endure. This chronic condition exacerbates the already difficult process of managing the disease by frequently causing emotions of isolation, worry, and uncertainty.

Individuals diagnosed with C. diff. colitis may suffer from increased mental distress, decreased adherence to treatment programmes, and a worse quality of life if they do not have access to sufficient support networks and community services. In addition, the absence of emotional support and direction can exacerbate feelings of helplessness and loneliness, which can have an adverse effect on one's physical and mental health.

The creation and application of community resources and support groups catered to the unique requirements of those suffering from C.

diff. colitis is the answer. Through these channels, people can connect with others going through similar struggles, exchange stories, get emotional support, and gain access to important data and services.

Putting this approach into practise entails starting and promoting online and in-person support groups where people can converse, exchange ideas, and get emotional support. Furthermore, assisting patients in gaining access to community resources including advocacy groups, educational materials, and mental health services can improve their emotional health and illness management.

There is evidence that those with C. diff. colitis who actively participate in support groups and make use of community resources have better emotional resilience, better disease management, higher treatment adherence, and a stronger sense of empowerment. These interventions may also help patients feel less distressed emotionally and build a network of support, which will enhance their general state of wellbeing.

Although community resources and support groups are the main focus here, it's crucial to recognise that other options, including individual counselling or therapy, might also be helpful for some people. However, support groups and community services give a special kind of emotional support that goes well with conventional therapeutic approaches because of the shared understanding and special sense of camaraderie they provide.

Support Groups: A Pillar of Emotional Resilience

Managing C. diff. colitis involves more than just physical combat; it also involves a major emotional and psychological war. In order to give people the emotional strength to traverse their health journey with courage and resilience, support networks and community resources are essential. These obstacles are inherent in chronic illness and are further exacerbated by emotions of uncertainty and isolation.

Support groups are essential for those managing C. diff. colitis because they help them become emotionally resilient. In order to help patients cope with the emotional intricacies of chronic disease, these groups provide a secure and supportive environment in which they can interact with others who have gone through comparable situations. These organisations foster a strong sense of strength and belonging in their members by offering a forum for candid conversation, insightful exchanges, and support from one another.

One of the main advantages of support groups is the understanding and validation that people get from their peers. The psychological toll of dealing with C. diff. colitis can frequently result in feelings of inferiority and loneliness since the difficulties encountered can not be easily comprehended by people who have not gone through such experiences. In a support group, people may open up about their challenges and victories without worrying about being judged. They will receive encouragement, affirmation, and understanding from people who genuinely understand the breadth of their experiences.

Support groups provide not just emotional but also a useful forum for exchanging useful knowledge and resources. Members can help each other navigate the intricacies of C. diff. colitis by exchanging insights regarding coping techniques, dietary suggestions, medication alternatives, and illness management tactics. They can do this by drawing from their collective experiences. These organisations also frequently give people access to advocacy projects, knowledgeable speakers, and instructional materials, arming them with essential information and tools to improve their health journeys.

Outside of support groups, community resources are essential for enhancing the emotional toughness of people with C. diff. colitis. These resources cover a broad range of services, such as advocacy groups, educational materials, and mental health help, all of which improve patients' overall wellbeing. Healthcare professionals and support group facilitators can ensure that patients have access to a variety of resources by facilitating connections between individuals and these resources. This allows them to provide patients with more emotional support and direction.

Incorporating community services and support groups into the illness management framework is a comprehensive strategy for tackling the psychological effects of C. diff. colitis. Healthcare professionals and leaders of support groups can create a holistic atmosphere of emotional support, empowerment, and resilience by identifying and attending to the complicated needs of their patients. This method emphasises the need of creating a supportive community for those with chronic illness and recognises that emotional well-being is a crucial aspect of total health.

The purpose of this section has been to explain the value of community services and support groups in addressing the emotional challenges associated with controlling C. diff. colitis. The information is intended to give readers a thorough grasp of how these tools can help patients develop emotional resilience and improve their general well-being. Please let me know whether you want me to go on or if there are any particular topics you would like me to look into more.

The Role of Family and Caregivers

Family and caregivers play a critical role in helping persons manage the challenges of C. diff. colitis by offering vital support, comprehension, and aid. In order to better understand the role that family and caregivers play in the treatment and welfare of people with C. diff. colitis, this section will go over their possible effects on quality of life in general, emotional support, and disease management.

Families and caregivers are included in the context of controlling C. diff. colitis in addition to the patient themselves. Understanding the intricate roles that family and caregivers play in helping patients and their support system deal with the obstacles that come with living with a chronic disease requires an appreciation of the multifaceted nature of these challenges.

The main problem here is the mental and physical toll that people with C. diff. colitis take, as well as the possible stress that it takes on caregivers and family members. For individuals in the support role, juggling the duties of caregiving with the requirement for empathy and emotional support creates a special challenge.

In the event that family members and caregivers fail to provide sufficient support and understanding, people with C. diff. colitis may suffer from increased emotional distress, decreased adherence to treatment regimens, and a poor quality of life. In addition, a deficiency in communication and support within the family unit can exacerbate the patient's feeling of isolation and negatively affect their physical and mental health.

The caregivers' and family members' active participation and support in the treatment and management of C. diff. colitis is the key to the solution. The care network may actively support the patient's resilience and overall well-being by acknowledging the critical role they play and giving them the resources and tools they need.

Putting this solution into practise entails encouraging open communication within the family, teaching family members and caregivers on the specifics of C. diff. colitis, and offering them the tools and resources they need to carry out their caring responsibilities with efficiency. Furthermore, putting them in touch with neighbourhood resources and support systems can improve their capacity to offer both practical help and emotional support.

Research indicates that family members' and caregivers' active participation and understanding can help people with C. diff. colitis feel more supported, manage their disease better, control their emotions more effectively, and stick to their treatment regimens. Additionally, by reducing emotional distress and creating a network of support for the patient and their support system, these therapies may enhance the patient's general state of wellbeing.

Although the role of family members and caregivers is the main focus here, it's vital to recognise that some people may also benefit from alternate alternatives like professional home care services or respite care. But in addition to professional care services, family members' and caregivers' special understanding and bond provide a different kind of emotional support.

The Integral Role of Family and Caregivers in C. Diff. Colitis Management

Managing C. diff. colitis is a journey that the individual does not travel alone. In order to provide the patient with the loving and supporting atmosphere that is necessary for both their physical and emotional well-being, family members and caregivers must be involved. Family and caregivers are essential to the care and management of C. diff. colitis because of their comprehension, help, and dedication.

The comprehension and compassion that people get from their loved ones is one of the main advantages of family participation. The psychological toll of caring for someone with C. diff. colitis can frequently result in feelings of vulnerability and alienation, thus having supportive and understanding family members and caregivers is crucial. They enhance the patient's emotional health and lessen the emotional strain brought on by a chronic illness by offering a nonjudgmental and encouraging environment.

Caregivers and family members are vital collaborators in the management of C. diff. colitis. Their assistance can greatly affect the patient's capacity to deal with the difficulties of the illness, from helping with everyday tasks to offering emotional support during times of illness. Furthermore, family members can actively participate in the efficient management of the condition and assist the patient in following their treatment plan if they are aware of the unique requirements and possible consequences associated with C. diff. colitis.

Making sure the patient's wants and concerns are met within the family unit requires effective communication. In order to guarantee that the patient's needs—both emotional and physical—are satisfied, family members and caregivers can serve as their advocates. Family members and caregivers can build a supportive network that enables the patient to actively engage in their care and voice their concerns and desires by encouraging an atmosphere of open communication and understanding.

Beyond the pragmatics of providing care, family members and caregivers enhance the general well-being of people with C. diff. colitis. They provide the patient with emotional stability, security, and reassurance that they are not travelling alone. Through the provision of companionship, reassurance, and a caring environment, they enhance the patient's emotional resilience and overall well-being, so augmenting their capacity to manage the arduousness of chronic illness.

Family members and caregivers can gain by interacting with community services and support networks that are suited to their individual requirements in addition to the help offered inside the family. These resources provide direction, instruction, and emotional support to caregivers, giving them the know-how and resources they need to carry out their duties and deal with the challenges of caring for someone who has C. diff. colitis.

The Family-Centered Approach to C. Diff. Colitis Care

Incorporating family members and caregivers into the illness management framework is a comprehensive strategy for tackling the psychological and physical effects of C. diff. colitis. Healthcare practitioners and support networks can cultivate a holistic environment of emotional support, empowerment, and resilience for patients and their support system by acknowledging their essential role and offering them the appropriate resources and assistance. This method emphasises the need of creating a supportive and understanding environment while acknowledging that the participation of family members and caregivers is crucial for the wellbeing of those managing chronic illness.

In conclusion, family members' and caregivers' participation in the treatment and management of C. diff. colitis is crucial for offering the patient practical help, understanding, and emotional support. The care network can positively impact a patient's resilience and overall well-being by acknowledging their essential role, encouraging transparent communication, and offering essential resources and support. This will ultimately improve the patient's capacity to confront chronic illness head-on with courage and strength.

Navigating Social Situations

This section aims to give advice on how to manage C. diff. colitis while interacting with others in social circumstances. It seeks to provide the reader with the knowledge and skills necessary to manage social situations and activities in a way that strikes a balance between their social and health-related obligations.

To accomplish the goal of treating C. diff. colitis while navigating social situations, no special materials are needed. Prior to participating in social activities, it is crucial to comprehend the person's health status, possible triggers, and personal restrictions.

Managing C. diff. colitis while navigating social situations requires a complete approach that takes into account the person's health needs, potential obstacles, and social interaction tactics. This entails expressing needs and boundaries, putting self-care techniques into practise in social situations, and comprehending how the illness affects social activities.

1. People must be fully aware of how C. diff. colitis may affect their capacity to participate in different social activities before engaging in social interactions. This entails identifying possible triggers, realising the importance of accessible restrooms, and appreciating how exhaustion and nutritional constraints affect social interactions.

2. Navigating social situations while controlling C. diff. colitis requires effective communication. People ought to have the confidence to express their demands and limitations to friends, relatives, and other acquaintances. This could entail communicating the necessity of knowing food constraints, the significance of easily accessible restrooms, and the possible influence of weariness on social events.

3. People with C. diff. colitis must prioritise self-care while they are in social settings. This can entail finding calm areas to retreat to during the day, having the right prescriptions or tools for managing symptoms on hand, and being aware of one's own energy levels when interacting

with others. Self-care techniques can assist people in properly managing their health demands while navigating social situations.

4. It's important to choose social activities that suit each person's tastes and demands in terms of health. This can entail selecting events that allow for flexibility and understanding for health-related needs, prioritising gatherings in familiar settings, and selecting activities that meet dietary restrictions.

- Tip 1:Plan Ahead: People should think about scheduling social events in advance to give themselves enough time to make the required arrangements and make sure that any prospective medical needs are taken care of.

- Tip 2:Advocate for Personal Needs: Whether it's food restrictions, bathroom accessibility, or the need for breaks, people should speak up for their own needs while they're in social situations.

Be careful: Overexertion: People with C. difficile colitis may experience worsening symptoms from physical strain and exhaustion, therefore they should use caution when participating in social activities.

In order to certify that they managed C. diff. colitis successfully while navigating social situations, people can evaluate their experiences using the following standards:

- Did their social contacts take into account their health needs?

- Did a good social experience stem from clear communication of needs and boundaries?

- Were self-care techniques applied, and did they improve the person's wellbeing when interacting with others?

If someone encounters obstacles or unforeseen problems when interacting with others, they may want to think about the following troubleshooting techniques:

- Reassessing Social Engagements: If people find that participating in a particular social activity presents problems on a regular basis, they should reconsider and look for alternatives that better suit their health requirements.

- Seeking Support: People can get help from family members, close friends, or medical professionals to deal with certain issues that come up in social situations.

Managing C. diff. colitis while navigating social circumstances calls for a deliberate and proactive strategy that puts the person's health requirements first while developing deep social ties. Through comprehension of the condition's effects, proficient communication of personal requirements, application of self-care techniques, and selection of appropriate social events, people can manoeuvre through social situations with assurance and regard for their welfare.

Inspirational Stories: Living With C. Diff

In my capacity as a physician and health and wellness coach, I have had the honour of hearing countless moving accounts of people who have persevered through the difficulties of having C. diff. colitis. These tales serve as potent monuments to the human spirit's ability to persevere in the face of misfortune, as well as shedding light on the daily challenges and victories faced by persons who have this illness. I hope to offer one such inspirational storey in this area that not only conveys the essence of living with C. diff. colitis but also provides important lessons and wisdom that readers can relate to on a worldwide basis.

As I made my way to the wellness centre, where I see my patients, the crisp autumn morning was complemented by the golden tones of the falling leaves. The calming sounds of a piano playing in the background welcomed me as I entered the peaceful area and created a serene mood. I had no idea that this day, which seemed routine at first, would turn into an unforgettable experience that would forever alter my path as a healthcare professional.

A woman seated in the waiting area's corner caught my eye among the serene atmosphere; her kind disposition and inviting smile suggested familiarity and comfort. The resilience and quiet fortitude in her eyes as she walked toward me told me a lot about the struggles and victories she has faced. Sarah, as she was called, was going to tell me a storey that would change my lifelong view of having C. diff. colitis.

Every word Sarah spoke as she started to describe her journey had a purpose and meaning. She talked about the initial shock and bewilderment that followed her diagnosis, the innumerable moments of hopelessness and doubt, and the steadfast will that kept her moving forward in the face of difficulty. Her storey came to life like a bravery and fortitude tapestry, with each strand creating a captivating storey of resiliency and hope.

Deep within Sarah's storey was a moving emotional landscape that spoke to the dread, uncertainty, and steadfast optimism that are shared by all people. She talked of the nights she spent struggling with the psychological and physical effects of her illness, the vulnerable moments that tried her resolve, and the steadfast support of her loved ones that helped her get through her darkest moments.

When Sarah's tale appeared to be reaching a point of no return, she revealed an unexpected twist that reflected the erratic nature of having C. diff. colitis. That was the moment she consciously chose to take back control of her life, to turn her challenges into learning experiences, and to adopt a holistic perspective on her health that went beyond the limitations of her illness.

Sarah's journey extended beyond the confines of personal experience, providing profound understandings of the human spirit's resiliency and the transformational potential of unshakable persistence. Her experience served as a reminder of the universal values of kindness, tenacity, and the unwavering pursuit of a meaningful life in spite of obstacles.

I was filled with a deep admiration for the human spirit's tenacity and the capacity for transformation that comes from adversity as Sarah came to the end of her storey. Her experience provided as a moving reminder that, even in the midst of adversity, there are seeds of resiliency and strength that are just waiting to be planted and grown.

By telling Sarah's tale, I wish to inspire readers to go on a path of self-awareness and empowerment, realising that every setback is a chance for improvement and every depressing moment serves as a spark for everlasting hope. We are encouraged to embrace the transforming potential of bravery and resilience via the prism of Sarah's experiences, and to develop a holistic perspective on well-being that takes the mind, body, and spirit into consideration.

This book's pages contain a tapestry of stories that shed light on what it's like to live with C. diff. colitis. Each storey offers a different viewpoint on resiliency, willpower, and the unwavering pursuit of a life full of vitality and purpose. These motivational stories act as beacons of hope, shedding light on the way to holistic health and providing insightful information that goes beyond personal experience.

As we delve into the profound wisdom and transforming potential that emerge from the lived experiences of those who have experienced the hardships of living with C. diff. colitis, I invite you to join me on a voyage of discovery and enlightenment in the chapters that follow. Together, let's explore the priceless lessons and revelations these tales have to give, paving the way for empowerment in the face of misfortune and comprehensive well-being.

Greetings from the threshold of these inspirational stories. May we accept the lessons they convey and come away enlightened, strong, and motivated to live a life full of energy, fortitude, and everlasting hope, no matter what challenges we face.

Milton Keynes UK
Ingram Content Group UK Ltd.
UKHW020642220124
436466UK00019B/900